Man, You Are Not Infertile

Veronica Anusionwu

The Lord's Word On Healing Series

The Lord's Word On Healing Publications

Copyright © Veronica Anusionwu
First published in 2000 by The Lord's Word On Healing Publications
The Lord's Word On Healing Ministries
P O Box 24604, London, E2 9XA

The right of Veronica Anusionwu to be identified as the author of the work has been asserted herein in accordance with the Copyright, Designs and Patents Act 1988.

All rights reserved. This book is sold subject to the condition that it shall not, by way of trade or otherwise, be lent, resold, hired out or otherwise circulated without the publisher's prior consent in any form of binding or cover other than that in which it is published and without a similar condition including this condition being imposed on the subsequent purchaser.

Books which I found useful for reference, are *Trying for a Baby* by Peter Moore (Lion Publishing) and the *BMA Family Health Encyclopedia* (Dorling Kindersley).

Unless otherwise indicated, bible quotes are from the *New International Version*, © 1973, 1978, 1984 by the International Bible Society, and used by kind permission of Hodder & Stoughton. Other editions quoted from include *The Amplified Bible, Old Testament*, © 1965, 1987 by the Zondervan Corporation; *The Amplified New Testament* © 1958, 1987 by the Lockman Foundation, used with kind permission, and *The King James Version of The Bible*.

ISBN 0-9532698-1 7
Scriptures in this book have been personalize to encourage individual application.

Printed and bound by Professional Book Supplies, Oxford, England

CONTENTS

Author's Preface

Introduction

Page

1. The role of the Holy Spirit in your life 1
2. Male Infertility 12
3. Azoospermia 21
4. Oligospermia 31
5. Impotence 39
6. Congenital Disorders 45
7. Idiopathic Infertility 59
8. Growth that affect the male reproductive organs 65
9. Men's ejaculation problems 70
10. What the Word of God can do in our life and body 81
11. How to avoid unnecessary test and treatment when having difficulty conceiving 85
12. The power of Gods word and the Power of your own words 88
13. Lets talk about faith 95
14. Giving 106
15. Major questions on infertility answered from the Bible 114
16. More questions on infertility answered from the Bible 134
17. The Father hood of God 154
18. Who is Jesus Christ? 158
19. Prayer Point 173
20. Daily Confessions 174

AUTHOR'S PREFACE

The Word of God is supernatural; mixing faith with the Word of God by speaking His words through your own mouth is a way of applying God's medicine. However, the Word of God only works by faith (simple belief that God meant what he said). If you do not have enough faith, go to your doctor to receive help, for God also uses doctors to perform miracles in people's lives and many lives are saved by doctors. The Word of God and the wisdom of your doctor will work togather to bless your life.

Our Lord Jesus Christ, after healing a man, sent him to go and have himself examined by his priest. (Priests were the doctors in those days; it was their duty to confirm the healing of the individual.) Luke 5: 14.

Do not throw your medicine away and rely on God's Word alone unless God tells you to do so.

Everything works by faith. See your doctor before you throw away your medication. Where there is no cure for your sickness then applying the Word of God by faith will surely bring about healing. When your faith grows you will be able to take God's Word for what your faith tells you, for God's Word can never fail. Use common sense and may God answer you in the day of trouble. (Psalms 20: 1)

NOTE

There are times you will read the word "man" in this book. Man here is not referring to gender as in male. But God call us all sons - both men and women. So, when you read, a righteous man, it is not referring to the "male" but to both sexes.

A note to doctors

I know the time will come when this book will come into the hands of those in the medical profession. God wants you to know that all medical problems are in his power. Where science has no answers you can use God's Word to make a difference. Every honest doctor will agree with me that the area of infertility has defied scientific research; this is because God has kept the final answer to Himself for his glory. Study this book carefully and question what is written and I pray that the Holy Spirit of God will help you to understand.

The will of man

God created each and every one of us with a will to choose. He gave us a will. God will never force anything on you or me, or ask us to do anything against our will. In his Word he has laid down the benefits of both good and evil but he advises us to choose good and do it. Our God will never do anything for anyone against their will. See the statements made by the Lord Jesus Christ like "if any man wills, let him come unto me and drink, if any man will open the door, I will come unto him and sup with him and him with me."

Man's consent is the first step into divine blessing. Christ is willing to help the helpless anywhere if the helpless are willing to acknowledge their helplessness and reveal a readiness to be guided. So today, I want you to know that to receive God's blessing, you must be willing and you must ask for it.

Deliberate repetitions

There are quite a few repetitions in this book, especially God's promises; why have I done this? Because whatever you read or hear again and again sticks in your memory. Why do you think CNN repeat the same news again and again. Because they want people to remember that news. So the repetitions are deliberate so that you will always remember God's promises to you.

God's method

> "For my thoughts are not your thoughts, neither are my ways your ways," declares the Lord. "As the Heavens are higher than the earth, so are my ways higher than your ways and my thoughts than your thoughts." Isaiah 55:8-9

Throughout this book, you will not read material anywhere about methods, because God does not work with methods. God will always manifest himself in your life because He always confirm his words, but the methods he has decided to use are always left to him. He will not allow us to reduce him to a recipe. Time and time again, I have seen God confirm His Word in the life of his people. The problem may be the same but the way He manifests Himself is always different in every case.

He will never show himself the same way twice. The Bible says, "His mercies are new every morning for great is his faithfulness." I have prayed for so many people, perhaps on the road as I go shopping or on an outing, and also many times in my own personal life, but he has never manifested Himself the same way twice. I have seen instant manifestation in prayers while other times there has been a waiting period before a visible manifestation is noticed. In all cases God hears the first prayers and answers them immediately but the final result and timing is best left to Him - the all-knowing and all-sufficient God. If you are trusting God's words, and His promise, hold fast; it may tarry, but it will surely come.

Women's confessions

These confessions which have placed in the relevant place throughout the book are general confessions which you should be able to confess every day until there is full manifestation of your desires. I have Kept them short, so that you can memorise them and keep confessing them until they grow and bear fruit in Jesus' name. Confess them as many times as you can, day and night. There are no side effects and it works. Remember to sit in a comfortable position and mediate on the promises of God you are confessing. God bless you.

INTRODUCTION

In the name that is above every name, the name of my Lord and Saviour, Jesus Christ, I welcome you to this book, part of *"The overcoming Infertility collection."* I am happy to present *The Lord's Word* to you. I am also happy to you tell you that Jesus loves you and wants you to know he is coming back again soon to take you home with him. Before He comes, He wants you to live a victorious life here on earth.

What a pleasure it has been for me just watching the great acts of our Lord and Saviour Jesus Christ come to life. Using things like bread and fish, saliva and mud, and water, we see the Bible miracles came alive once again to heal and restore us thousands of years after they were recorded. What about the story of David and Goliath written at least three to four thousand years ago? Yet it has never lost its power. Once again it appears here to bring healing and hope to those who think their victory is based on numbers rather than on God.

I am thrilled to be the vessel through which the Holy Spirit has brought about these books. The problem of infertility in our generation is not a small one. Over a hundred million couples are estimated to face this problem world-wide. Yet in the very heart of God is an overwhelming desire to bless all human beings with children. Today, I desire that we look away from the inadequacies of our medical researches to the banquet of rich food prepared for us by almighty God. Jesse Duplantis said about his trip to Heaven in his book (*Close Encounters Of The God Kind*):

> "I saw new lives of little babies singing and flying around God's throne. It seemed to be that babies just came out of the breath of God. They looked like they were wearing night gowns.
> They flew into the presence of Jehovah. I realised they were new souls who came from the thoughts of God. God thinks kids. Now I know why those new-born babies are

so precious. Babies are gifts given to us directly from the throne of God."

I personally believe this is true, for God has given me a tiny glimpse into His love and desire for mankind - a desire to bless us with all that we ever desire or need.

Today, I invite you to come and partake of this great banquet prepared by almighty God. This book you are holding is a prayer; this book has been born in the ovens of prayer. I have prayed, I have cried and studied hard to be able to write this book. I have received so many miracles already that if you will fix your faith, babies are going to just come - Bam! Bam! Bam! It will amaze you. If you will dare to fix your faith (trust) in Jesus and His promise that is written for you, you will receive all your heart's desire so that your joy may be complete.

Never in my life have I known such love as the love that flows from the heart of God to all mankind. Reach out in trust like a little baby and receive it.

I have written these books to bring you joy and happiness in your home because that's what Jesus has commanded me to do. In this book I have written everything that you need to know about infertility, from the Bible, from the very heart of God. God has promised to bless you with all that you need so that your joy will be complete. I have written all the Lord has told me to write to His beloved men and women and I stand upon these promises because Jesus Christ is no mere man. No mere human could promise to solve all the problems of the world. But in His promise that he is able to meet all our needs, he proves once and for all that He alone is the great creator of the Heavens and the earth and all that is in it.

Today I encourage you to receive the truth written down and in doing so you will be mightily blessed. God Bless You And Remember Jesus Loves You.

Chapter One

The Role of The Holy Spirit In Your Life

In the Name that is above every name, the Name of our Lord and Saviour Jesus Christ, I welcome you to this book, and I would like to tell you this, *"Jesus loves you and cares about you."*

My question to you today is this, "Do you know the Holy Spirit?" Consider if your answer to this question is no, then allow me to introduce you to Him, if your answer is yes I encourage you to read this chapter and get to know Him even more. He is the One Who wrote this book, to the *"glory of Jesus Christ,"* so that the blessings and goodness of God will come to you.

He is the One Whom Jesus left on earth for us. For the Lord Jesus Christ, before He left to go back to the Father, promised us this:

> I will ask the Father, and he will give you another Counsellor to be with you for ever - the Spirit of truth. The world cannot accept him, because it neither sees him nor knows him. But you know him, for he lives with you and will be in you. I will not leave you as orphans. I will come to you." (John 14: 16-18)

From this passage you can see that the Holy Spirit is already here on earth with us. isn't it possible to have Him with us and yet totally miss His presence and His love, because we have not taken the time to find out Who He is.

You say I call Him *"He"*. Yes, the Holy Spirit of God is a person. He is not a mere influence or force coming from God. He is a real person. Jesus said, *"...that he may abide with you."* He is not an it. He is a real person. He is not just a power. He is a person.

The Holy Spirit speaks (Revelation 2: 11). A force cannot speak to people. The Holy Spirit comforts people-In John 14:16-18- He is described as the comforter. In Ephesians 4: 30 we see that the Holy Spirit can be grieved. A force cannot be grieved.

From these few Bible verses, you can see that the Holy Spirit is a person: In Romans 15: 30 -The Apostle Paul refers to the love of the Holy Spirit as the love of Christ.

Before I continue, I beseech you brethren for the love of Christ, and the love of the Holy Spirit.

Have you ever thought of the love of the Holy Spirit? The love of God the Father is the love of the Holy Spirit - "The love of the Spirit is the love of Jesus Christ, which caused Him to leave His throne in Heaven and come down to earth to dwell in the midst of selfish, sinful men. It is the love that led Him to bleed to death on the Cross; having loved His own, He loved them to the end. For God so loved the world that He gave His only Son. (John 3: 16).

That is the unconditional love of God, without which the whole world would have been lost. It is the love of the Son, which no human language is able to express. It is deeper than the deepest sea. Yet today, I will say this to you, the love of the Father would have been in vain; the self-sacrificing love of Jesus Christ of no purpose, if it had not been for that great, patient, infinite love of the blessed Holy Spirit working in our heart. The working of the Trinity is the mystery of the Gospel of Jesus Christ. It is better to accept it than to try to figure it out, for only in Heaven will we clearly understand it all. Take what you have and apply it and let it work for you.

My personal relationship with the Holy Spirit

I would like to share my testimony with you about the Holy Spirit, and the reason why I choose to start the first chapter of this book with the Holy Spirit.

I met the Holy Spirit for the first time in August 1992, the day I gave my heart to the Lord. After that service, I went to the bookshop of that church and I bought three books that laid a total foundation for my Christian walk. One of those books was *Good Morning Holy Spirit* by Benny Hinn. In it he shared with us about his relationship with the Holy Spirit and how he found out the Holy Spirit was a person, and what he did to establish his relationship with Him.

Being a new Christian and having no spiritual experience, I did what Benny had done. The next morning, I selected a corner in my daughter's room, put a rug there, sat down and I said, *"Good Morning Holy Spirit."* Immediately I said it, I felt His power and presence on me, and I started weeping. It was the most wonderful experience of my life. I then knew for myself that the Holy Spirit was a real person. I also learnt that the Holy Spirit was my Teacher, that if my Christian walk was going to be fruitful and successful, I was to know the Holy Spirit as a person.

Well, not only did I get to know Him as a person, I fell in love with Him. He started to teach me things from the Bible, and show me all that Jesus had done for me, and how the blood of Jesus had paid for all my sins, and provided for all I will ever need in life.

Within three weeks of knowing the Holy Spirit, something happened inside of me. I could no longer stand to see suffering or anyone sick. I started to pray for sick people on the road or in the bus, and God just healed them there on the spot. Seeing these miracles my faith in God grew and so did my desire to reach out for those in need. The Holy Spirit would wake me up at night to go and pray for someone, and He would heal them.

Within a period of six months of knowing the Holy Spirit, He had taught me so much. I can say to the glory of God that, because of my relationship with the Holy Spirit, I did not require any counselling or have any need to run up and down looking for people to answer my questions, because whatever problems I faced, He always dealt with them and answered all my questions, and directed me in all my ways. Everything I did, I consulted the Holy Spirit and He directed me.

Remember the Bible says, "In all your ways acknowledge the Lord, and He will direct your path." (Proverbs 3: 6) This is exactly my principle for walking with the Lord. I can boldly tell you that God has been faithful and true to His Word. The Holy Spirit has been my Comforter and my God. Throughout the years I have walked with the Lord, He has been true to His promise, he has guided me in all my ways and directed my footsteps. I can boldly declare to you that God is true and His Word perfect.

I have taken time to share just a little bit of my experience, to encourage you to get to know Him for yourself. This book is His work.

Every thing written in this book are only as a result of His help.

He gives faith

He gives faith as a gift (I Corinthians 12: 9). We may not know how He creates faith, but I think it is enough to know that He does.

Faith is one of His gifts even as faithfulness is part of His fruit. An example from the Bible is that of Stephen and Barnabas. They were men full of faith and the Holy Spirit (Acts 6: 5, Acts 11: 24); from this we can see that a special manifestation of faith is a result of fullness of the Holy Spirit.

The Holy Spirit creates the faith in our heart, through which we receive salvation. One of the ways He imparts faith in our hearts is through those that belong to Christ like Apostles, Prophets, Evangelists, Pastors and Teachers, etc. The Holy Spirit convicts the person of their sin as the word of God is proclaimed and creates in their heart the need for the Saviour.

To write this book has taken great faith on my part. And I tell you the truth, I would never have attempted it, if not for the fullness of God's Holy Spirit, and His faithfulness to me, and because of my love for my Lord Jesus, and my commitment to obey and serve Him. These are some of the benefits of knowing the Holy Spirit.

Physical life

The Holy Spirit is the One Who gives life, both spiritual and physical life. Before God could create anything on earth, the Holy Spirit was already there to breath life into whatever God said.

> Now the earth was formless and empty. Darkness was over the surface of the deep, and the Spirit of God was hovering over the waters. And God said, Let there be light, and there was light. (Genesis 1: 1-3)

The Bible says in the Psalms that when God sends His Spirit, that is when we are created.

The Holy Spirit is the One Who creates life. The Spirit gives life (John 6: 63). Every life on earth today is given by the Holy Spirit. Those of you who desire to have children, it is the Holy Spirit Who will give that life to the child in your womb. We hear the angel of God telling Mary:

> The Holy Spirit will come upon you, and the power of the Most High will overshadow you. (Luke 1: 35)

So it is the Spirit that gives life to a baby in the womb. Even when we become pregnant, no one can claim knowledge of the exact time conception took place. All these things are secret things that belong to God, but the important thing I want you to know is this, the Holy Spirit is the giver of life.

The Holy Spirit gives life to our mortal bodies (Romans 8: 11), which means that any death that exists in your body, can be resurrected by the Holy Spirit living inside you.

Spiritual life

It is the Holy Spirit who gives spiritual life. He is the One Who bestows it. He tends and nurtures that life. No man can redeem himself or sanctify himself. All these are works of the Holy Spirit. He works in us, creating in our heart the desire for a Saviour, leading us patiently to Jesus, and sustaining us.

A man can achieve only so much in his own strength, he can acquire knowledge by diligent study, but he cannot win for himself the life which is from God. Eternal life.

The modern man will say today, *"Seek your own salvation. All ways lead to God. We believe in freedom of religion."* Some will not direct their children in the way of God. "Oh, when he grows up, he will choose which God he wants to serve, because these days there are too many gods." But this new gospel of the modern man only leads to disappointment. If man could save himself, God would not have sacrificed His only Son for our redemption.

Salvation is a gift from God. The Holy Spirit alone can do what no human can do for us. He is the giver of life. "Not by works of righteousness which we have done, but according to His mercy He saved us by the washing of regeneration and renewing of the Holy Ghost. (Titus 3: 5)

Helping our weakness

The Bible says in Romans 8: 26 that the Holy Spirit helps our weaknesses. In our prayer we often find that we do not know what to pray. Many of you reading this book might never even have prayed before, but the Holy Spirit will teach you how to pray, according to the will of God. He will show you what you need and what to do in every situation you face. He creates in our heart a longing after more prayer. He glorifies

Christ. He shows us His glory. If you don't know how and what to pray, ask the Holy Spirit to help you pray. He will pray through you. You will have answers to prayers that will amaze you. You will experience that "He is able to do immeasurably more than all we can ask or imagine, according to the power that is at work within us." (Ephesians 3: 20)

The Holy Spirit sheds the love of God in our hearts (Romans 5: 5)

A lawyer may be very able in his profession without necessarily loving his clients. A doctor can have success without loving his patients. A businessman may prosper without loving his customers. But you can never be a worker of Christ without a deep passion for lost souls. Love alone is the key to the hearts of all men. Even the hardest heart cannot, in the long run, resist the influence of love. Why did our Lord leave His home in Heaven to come to this sinful earth? Was it not His great compassion and love which led Him to die on the Cross of Calvary?

> Greater love hath no man than this, that he lay down his life for his friend. (John 15: 13)

One day Paul was asked what drove him from land to land, from city to city. "After they stoned you at Lystra, why do you preach the same Gospel in Derbe? Why are you exposing yourself to many dangers?" His answer was simple and plain: *"The love of Christ compels us."* (2 Corinthians 5: 14)

When the Lord showed me my vision and the work he called me to do, these were His words to me: *"Veronica, to do this work, you will have to love everybody."* My first question to Him was, *"Lord, how is that possible?"* He told me it could be done by the Holy Spirit. Today, six years down the road, I can say to the glory of God that I am learning, day by day, to love everybody. When I look at people, all I see is Jesus Christ, the One Who created them in His image. I try to look away from their weaknesses, because I have a bag full of mine as well, but I look at them through the eyes of God, the eyes and heart full of love for all mankind.

Many of you reading this book may not know how to love God, because no one ever told you, but I can guarantee you, if you ask the Holy Spirit, he will shed the love of Christ abroad in your heart.

The Holy Spirit gives freedom

The Bible says, "Where the Spirit of the Lord is there is liberty." (II Corinthians 3: 17) There are many people today, even among the Christians, who are still bound by one thing or another, because they do not have the Spirit of Christ in them.

One day in a Sunday School Class, a teacher asked a boy if he could break a piece of thread. The boy smiled, "Of course I can do that." The teacher placed the boy in the middle of the class and had him bound with that thread until he could not move. The thread was stronger than the boy.

> But every man is tempted when he is drawn away of his own lust and enticed, then when lust hath conceived, it bringeth forth sin and sin, when it is finished, bringeth forth death. (James 1: 14)

The beginning of sin lies in our thoughts. We all have sinful imaginations, then a moment comes when we do not resist any more. The sinful thoughts become sinful acts, and when often repeated, become a sinful habit. Then the soul is bound. We may have life, but lack the freedom.

Take an example, the lion caged up in a zoo has life, but has no freedom. He wrestles in vain to be free. He beats the iron bars in vain. He can never free himself. Someone else must give him freedom.

Are you bound today? - by sickness, demonic oppression, etc? Then this is Who you need - the Holy Spirit of God, because, where the Spirit of God is, there is liberty. Be filled with the Spirit of God and all chains will fall. Do you want to be free, free from pain and sin? Do you really long for freedom? Then come to Jesus. He can help you.

How can I receive the Holy Spirit?

The world cannot receive the Holy Spirit, because they do not know Him. (*John 14: 17*). He comes to the children of God. The fullness and power of the Holy Spirit is for all God's children.

Those who, after reading this book, decide to invite the Lord into their heart to be their Saviour, will also receive the Holy Spirit. The fact that you have gone to church since you were born, does not help at all. You must personally invite Jesus to come into your heart and be your Lord and Saviour, then the Holy Spirit comes too. When He comes He helps you to grow spiritually, teaches you Who Jesus is, what your rights as a child of God are, and gives you all the benefits mentioned in the Word of God.

Have you received the Holy Spirit?

In concluding this chapter on the Holy Spirit, I would like to share a sad story with you, which had a happy ending and I leave you today with this question. *What will you do with the Holy Spirit?*

The story of Mary

This is the story of Mary who was a widow. After a short, happy married life, her husband died, leaving her with their only son, Andrew. She was a poor widow, but all she wished was for her Andrew to have a good education. She worked day and night. No sacrifice was too much to make for her Andrew, and the son rewarded her by his hard work.

Eventually Andrew completed his education and became a famous lawyer. He moved to a big city, and then his mother seldom saw him. His profession took up all his time.

After some time, Andrew married a girl from a rich family, and after this event, his mother did not see him at all.

Shall I tell you why? I am almost ashamed to say it. This great lawyer had a narrow soul. He was ashamed to confess to his wife his humble beginnings. He feared his wife would be ashamed of his mother. Yet deep down in his heart, Andrew longed for his mother. He had not forgotten her love and care. His longing for his mother finally led him to speak to his wife.

This is what Andrew told his wife. "You know my dear, how servants in the country are different from those in the city. At home we had a faithful maid. When I was sick, she watched over me through many long nights. Had she not cared so faithfully for me, you would never have known me. Up there in the attic, we have a little room, which is not used. If you agree, we will send for dear Mary to come and live with us."

With joy, the young wife gave her consent to the kind plan of her husband. So Andrew sat down and wrote a long letter to his mother. He told her of his wife and how she would not understand that his mother was so plain and simple, and begged her to come to him, but not to tell anyone that she was his mother.

Do you think the mother sent the letter back, outraged? Andrew certainly would have deserved it if she had. A father might have done so, but what would a mother's heart not do in order to be near her son?

She came: a plain little woman. She was introduced to the lawyer's wife: "This is the faithful Mary." From that moment on, Mary lived in the room in the attic.

Humbly, Mary settled down in her new home. When his young wife went out, Andrew sneaked up to his mother's room. Then he would talk to her of his childhood and those hours were the greatest joy of his mother's life.

Nobody else noticed Mary's presence in the house. The dear old Mary remained hidden in her room. Only once, on her arrival, had she been into the beautiful rooms of her son's home. She lived in his home, but only in the attic.

Before I continue this story, I just want to tell you that is how many of us have treated the Holy Spirit of God. He has been with us all the time, but we have locked Him up in our attic. We are too ashamed to bring Him out. Our fancy friends would not understand. Our beautiful wives or husbands will not love us any more, so we have turned out the One Who is like a loving and kind mother to us; the One Who is our Comforter, our Guide; the One Who is supposed to help us when we are weak; the One Who is supposed to teach us all things. We have turned Him out and locked Him in the attic. And because we have done this, we are now left to struggle and suffer. There is no victory in our lives, no wisdom, no Godly knowledge, because, you see, it is the Holy Spirit Who is supposed to teach us all things. While we struggle because of lack of power in our lives, the Holy Spirit sleeps in our attic. What are we going to do next?

I continue Mary's story. True love cannot be deceived. The young wife soon noticed that something was depressing her husband. She asked him, and he told her the truth, that Mary was his mother.

The young wife was so sad and hurt very deeply. She asked her husband, *"How could you believe that I was so narrow-minded?"*

Many of the people you are ashamed to share Jesus Christ with or the Holy Spirit with, are looking for Him. They know something is missing in their lives. So don't think people are so narrow-minded.

Hand in hand, Andrew and his young wife went up to the attic room. His wife took the old woman's hand and pressed her fresh young cheeks against the old one, and said softly, "Mother!!!" The young couple knelt before the old mother and asked for her forgiveness.

Then they led Mary downstairs and the prettiest and sunniest room, in the house, was given her. And from that moment happiness returned into the home.

Once again, I would like to ask you two questions: *"Have you received the Holy Spirit? What will you do with the Holy Spirit?"*

Receiving Him is welcoming Him into your life, into your home, giving Him His rightful place as the One Who is called to take you by the hand, and teach you all things, guide you into all truth. He must have His rightful place in your lives or else you can never have the victory God intended for you to have.

The Bible says, "As many as received Him, He gave them power to become the sons of God." This is the beginning of the Christian life. It begins with receiving and not giving, and continues like that to the end. The father gives, the child accepts. For our lives to have meaning we must put the Holy Spirit in His rightful place. If we fail to do that we will never taste true victory in this world.

One of the most powerful acts of the Holy Spirit was the virgin birth. The birth of our Lord Jesus was a miracle.

> The Angel of God appeared to Mary, and told her these words, "Do not be afraid, Mary, you have found favour with God. You will be with child and give birth to a Son, and you are to call His Name, Jesus. He will be great and will be called the Son of the Most High."
>
> Mary asked, "How will this be, since I am a virgin?"
>
> The Angel answered, "The Holy Spirit will come upon you, and the power of the Most High will overshadow you. So the Holy One to be born will be called the Son of God. (Luke 1: 30, 34-35)

Many people doubt the *virgin birth*. This has robbed them of God's blessing. For me, this passage of scripture has established me for ever in the kingdom of God. I totally trust the Holy Spirit. If my Lord and Saviour Jesus, Who was at the right hand of God, trusted the Holy Spirit to bring Him down to earth and conceive Him in the womb of a virgin, then for me there is no reason why I cannot trust the Holy Spirit totally. Try trusting Him and see what He will do. For many of you, men and women, who desire to conceive, this is the Person Who is the giver of life. No one can stop the Holy Spirit, when He decides to move.

The Bible says in Psalm 104: 30, "When you [God] send your Spirit, they are created." Wherever the Spirit of God is there is creativity, because He is the giver of life. He is the One that creates the words that come from our lips, the words that are conceived by the Word of God.

I want to encourage you to know the Giver of life Himself.
Receive the Holy Spirit.

How do I receive him?

Invite Jesus into your life as the Lord of your life. When Jesus is the Lord of your life the Holy Spirit also comes. Develop your relationship with the Holy Spirit by talking to Him and sharing things with Him as you would share with a spouse. You will be amazed to see what you will discover. The Holy Spirit is a *real person. God bless you as you pursue this relationship.*
Your prayer

Sweet Holy Spirit! I have read about You. I never knew Who you were or that I could have a personal relationship with You. Today I know for sure that you are a Person and that you are my Teacher and my friend. Take me by the hand and lead me. I don't even know which way to go or what to do, but I belive and trust that from to day You will lead and guide me in all my ways in Jesus name. Thank You for loving me and caring for me and from today teach me how to love You in Jesus name I pray. Amen.

Chapter Two

Male Infertility

Male infertility - what words! I always thought infertility was a woman's problem until the Lord called me to write this book. I then discovered that infertility affects men as well as women; thirty per cent of cases are caused by male factors and thirty per cent by female factors while in the remaining forty per cent of cases, infertility is due to both partners.

Who is an andrologist?

I came across the word *andrologist* for the first time when doing the research for this book. Who is an andrologist? He is a person who specialises in male reproductive disorders. I also learnt that this area of medicine was only started in the 70s. Until then no one thought anything could go wrong with a man's reproductive system. Thank God today we have more andrologists working to help identify the problems of infertility in couples' lives - knowing exactly who is to be treated whether it be the man or woman.

Men hate sperm tests

I also discovered that men really hate undergoing any test to find out if infertility can be attributed to them. The test a man undergoes is a simple test which involves taking a fresh sample of semen to a hospital or clinic; there it is examined under a microscope to check that the sperm are moving properly and how well they swim through viscous solutions. A man will allow his wife to go through so many complicated test, before agreeing to have this simple semen test.

I also found out that a man's image is so wrapped up in his sexuality that the thought that not being able to father a child might be his fault is unacceptable and difficult to contemplate; this is best described in the Bible by Jacob who said these words about his sexuality: "Reuben, you are my first-born, my might, the first sign of my strength, achievement, accomplishment..." This feeling is totally right and every man should feel that way because God created man to reproduce. The Bible says, "God created man in his image." "God then blessed them and said, 'Be fruitful and increase in number.'" (Genesis 1: 27-28) God's main reason for creating man was for him to reproduce. The Bible says: "Adam lay with his wife and she became pregnant." (Genesis 4:1) That is the desire of every man - to lie with his wife and for her to become pregnant. No long stories, no unnecessary sperm test, that is the desire of every man; that is why men hate going through all those tests. They are the seed of Adam, they just want to lay with their wives and get on with the business. God did not promise them unnecessarily long sperm tests, just that they should lie with their wives, increase and fill the earth; that is God's main purpose for creating man. That is God's desire for every man.

In the world today, we find that this position has changed. Many things have affected the fertility of so many men. Some men have even being told after many medical tests that they can never be fathers in their lifetime. These reports have made many men lose hope of ever becoming fathers; the sad thing about this is that even born-again Christian men accept this situation. It is sad to see many Christian men who have lost hope and lost faith that they can ever become fathers, but I thank God for His Word and His promises which can never fail those who put their hope in His unfailing love and faithfulness.

God's will for man

Taking a journey through the pages of the Bible under the guidance of the Holy Spirit, I am going to show you what God's perfect will for man is. Starting from the day God created man, His will for man was made clear, "Be fruitful and increase..." (Genesis 1:28) From the day of man's creation to this day, God's desire for man is for fruitfulness and for his increase.

I will be repeating God's promises of fruitfulness on several occasions as they appear in the Bible. I want you to know these repetitions are not mine, they are not coming from me. God spoke at different times and to different prophets repeating these promises, because He did not want man to forget what His perfect will for him is.

A short time after this command, Adam knew his wife, Eve, and she gave birth to Cain and Abel. This was the fulfilment of God's command and we see how man started to multiply and life continued on earth.

There came a time when man fell out of the will of God and God destroyed the earth with a flood; however, the Bible records that God found Noah to be faithful among the people of that time and God started again with him. "Noah was a righteous man, blameless among the people of his time, and he walked with God." (Genesis 9 : 9) When the world was destroyed by flood, God started again with Noah - this is God's command to Noah: "Be fruitful and increase in number and fill the earth." (Genesis 9 : 1) God repeats this command a second time to Noah: "As for you, be fruitful and increase in number, multiply on the earth and increase upon it." (Genesis 9 : 7) This is still God's plan for man - increase.

God calls Abraham

When God called Abraham in Genesis 12 : 2, Abraham did not have any children and Abraham cried out to God: "O Sovereign Lord, what can you give me since I remain childless and the one who will inherit my estate is Eliezer of Damascus?" (Genesis 15 : 2) But note God's promise to Abraham: "I will make you into a great nation and I will bless you."

God again continued this promise to Abraham: "I will make you fruitful; I will make nations of you and kings will come from you." (Genesis 17: 6) God then manifested His promise to Abraham and the Bible records: "The Lord did for Sarah what he had promised; Sarah became pregnant and bore a son to Abraham in his old age." (Genesis 21: 1) Here we see God's faithfulness and promise being fulfilled.

Abraham became the father of Isaac and when Isaac was forty years old, he married Rebekah. "Isaac prayed to the Lord on behalf of his wife, because she was barren. The Lord answered his prayer and his wife became pregnant." (Genesis 25 : 19) Why did God answer him? God had earlier made a promise of fruitfulness to Abraham. God again pledged His covenant to Isaac: "I swore to your father, Abraham, I will make your descendants as numerous as the stars in the sky and through your offspring all nations on earth will be blessed, because Abraham obeyed me and kept my requirements, my commands, my decrees and my laws." (Genesis 26: 4-5)

God spoke these words to Isaac to remind him of God's promise to his father.

We see this promise also reiterated in the life of Jacob who was Isaac's son. Jacob had gone away to live in Paddan Aram with his uncle, Laban, and while there he married and had so many children, that when he returned home his brother Esau looked up and saw the women and children who were with him and asked him, "Who are these with you?" Jacob answered, "They are the children God has graciously given your servant." (Genesis 33: 5) If you continue through the Bible, this promise of fruitfulness is carried through to the end. We read about the descendants of Abraham being too numerous to be counted; the Bible records: "Who can count the dust of Jacob or number the fourth part of Israel?" (Numbers 23: 10) The man who made this statement saw a multitude of people too numerous to be counted by anyone. Moses, the servant of God, spoke to God's people and said to them: "The Lord your God has increased your numbers so that today you are as many as the stars in the sky. Even also may the Lord, the God of your fathers, increase you a thousand times and bless you as he promised." (Deuteronomy 1: 10-11) God's promise to His people always includes their children. "Teach your children and tell them to teach their own children also, so that it may go well with you and your children after you." (Deuteronomy 4: 40)

God's desire is for every God-fearing man to leave children as witnesses who will declare God's goodness to the world long after their fathers may have died.

God's promise is to show love to a thousand generations of those who love him and keep his commandments. (Deuteronomy 5: 10) This statement is quite clear - the guarantee comes from God Himself, an assurance of a thousand generations of children; what a mighty God we serve. God's plan for man continues in Deuteronomy 6: 5-7 - "Love the Lord your God with all your heart and with all your soul and with all your strength. These commands are to be upon your heart, impress them on your children. Talk about them when you sit at home and when you walk down the road and when you lie down and when you get up." We can clearly see that God's desire is to bless us with children to whom we can teach His ways so that they in turn will teach their own children and others; all His blessings are tied up in our children. He promises us this: "He will love you and bless you and increase your numbers. He will bless the fruit of your womb, you will be blessed more than any other people, none of your men or women will be childless." (Deuteronomy 7: 14) What does none mean? None means None; that is God's Word, and God and His Word never changes.

If I were to continue throughout the pages of the Bible you will see that throughout His Word, God's perfect will for His children, for mankind, is fruitfulness, to increase in all areas, to have children and even more children to fill your life with happiness and joy.

Question

Why has this position changed today? Why is it that so many men are now becoming infertile and some are even giving up totally? One of the reasons for this is ignorance. People don't really know what God's perfect will is for them.

For every man, infertility brings him to the question, "Am I still a man?" That leads in turn to self-denial, anger, depression and painful moments - moments when fear of lack of success grips, feelings of inadequacy, loss of dignity and many other emotional upset that men go through.

I however want to bring you to my Lord and Saviour, Jesus Christ who said: "If you abide in me, and my word abides in you, you will bear much fruit. I am the vine and you are the branches. If a man remains in me and I in him, he will bear much fruit; apart from me you can do nothing." (John 15: 5) God has promised us that if we abide in Christ, we will bear fruit. Fruit in the scriptures can be interpreted as children. This applies to both physical and spiritual fruit-bearing. If we are in Christ, we are meant to be producers, fountains of life, drawing life from the tree and bringing forth fruit from the life received from the tree itself.

Grafted onto Christ, we are in Him like the branches are in the vine. We begin to participate in the divine life, and all that is dead in us is transfigured, made alive. I just apply this to infertility or barrenness and now boldly declare that no Christian who is serving God, nor any man who chooses to go with Christ after reading this book will remain childless. The Bible says: "God always leads us to victory through our Lord Jesus Christ." (1 Corinthians 15: 57) What does victory mean? It means to overcome an enemy or succeed in a struggle or endeavour. The Bible says that through Christ we will overcome all our enemies and succeed in all our endeavours. When God says all, He means all. Please don't try to reason yourself out of a miracle by thinking that in your situation it can't happen. The Bible has promised us victory in all we do, it promises much fruit in Christ. It promises us that none shall be barren in His house and God really means it. God said that His covenant with us is one of life and not death. So from what you have read so far, you can see that God's perfect will for mankind is to multiply and replenish the earth. He created the man with the most powerful equipment, the male reproductive organ, designed to produce life.

Authority and command

One interesting aspect of infertility that the Holy Spirit taught me about is the place of command and authority. This is to encourage you to hold on to the commands of God because they cannot fail.

What is to command?

To command means to direct authoritatively. Who gives this command? Someone in authority always gives a command to some one under that authority. That command, once given, must be carried out without any questions asked. Questions may be asked after the command has been carried out.

What is authority?

A person in authority is described as an individual cited or appealed to as an expert. Authority is the power to require and receive submission, the right to expect obedience, power to influence or command; a right granted by somebody in authority; a person in command; a government body

From this dictionary description we see God as the highest authority requiring our obedience and submission. God as the creator of the universe gave these commands to man: "Be fruitful and increase over the earth." God therefore authorised man - gave him legal power or empowered him to multiply and increase on the earth.

A commanding authority must as a rule provide all the essential equipment needed to enable his subjects to carry out the command given without hardship or difficulty. Even the Bible asks this question in I Corinthians 9: 7: "Who serves as a soldier at his own expense?" The answer is nobody. When a nation sends men to war they must provide their fighting men with guns, bullets, food, warm cloths, uniforms, medical care and everything the solider requires for the success of that assignment; and so it is in the spiritual realm. God who created us and commanded us to multiple has no choice but to provide us with all that we need to accomplish this command.

As you can see man had no choice in this matter; he could not choose. God commanded man to multiply and increase, so God must provide for the man all he will need to fulfil this assignment.

All his reproductive organs must be working perfectly and be in good order. If anything is missing, God as the commanding authority has the power and the ability to fix it. You may say that God was only speaking to Adam and Eve. No! when God spoke to them, you and I were in seed form in the bodies of these people. "Adam named his wife Eve because she would become the mother of all the living." (Genesis 3: 20)

The Bible says it is: "through one man that God created all nations of men [women]." (Acts 17: 26) Even Eve was taken from the man. God works in "potential" principles. In one man He packaged the seed to populate the whole world. Medically, it is a fact that a man produces in his testes about ten million sperm cell a day. This figure alone is enough to populate the whole world in just six months, yet all that is needed to make a baby is just one sperm. So there is no doubt that we all were in Adam the day God created him. If only one man in six months can provide enough sperm to populate the whole world then the Bible account is to be relied upon totally; from one man God created the whole nation of men. (Acts 17: 26)

Right now, all the children you desire are locked up inside you; you need the Word of God, spoken out of your mouth in faith (trust), to bring those children out, according to the power that works within you.

Doctors may have told you, "It is impossible; you can't father children." Whose report will you believe? God says that you can, while man says that you can't. Choose today for yourself what you will believe. Remember this command: "Be fruitful, increase and replenish the earth." (Genesis 1: 28) This is God's command to you.

Effects and the importance of God's commands

God's Word cannot be bound

One thing about God's commandments is that they are boundless. The Bible says: "God's commandments are boundless." (Psalms 119: 96) What does boundless means? It means His commands cannot be limited by any circumstances or lack of. He who created the universe and created you and me, gave us His commandment to "multiply", have children;

nothing in your life is suppose to stop you from fulfilling this call. What you lack is insufficient reason, be that male factors like low sperm count, no sperm count, or congenital disorder; nothing is supposed to stop you.

Where any lack exists you have every right to ask God to meet that need. You may ask me where I can see God. God himself invited us to "...come boldly before the throne of mercy that we may receive mercy and find grace to help us in our time of need." (Hebrews 4: 16) God even went further and invited us to come and reason together with Him. This is an open invitation from the creator of the universe to His children. (Isaiah 1: 18) God invites us to come and reason with Him.

God is ready to talk to you any day, any time, anywhere, if you are ready. If you are sincere and desire the truth, God will surely meet with you and reason with you. He will answer your deepest questions and solve the problems nobody can solve. He will give you the desires of your heart in Jesus' name. Remember that God's commandments are boundless.

All God's commandments are trustworthy

All God's commandments are trustworthy. (Psalms 119: 86) This means you can totally rely on them, you can totally depend on them, you can totally put your confidence in them, because they are honest and true. God alone will never lie to you or deceive you.

God's commandments give wisdom

All God's commandments will make you wiser than your enemy, amongst which is infertility (Psalms 119: 98), for God's commandments are ever with you.

When infertility stares you in the face, you can say to it, "Because of God's commandments, I am going to have that child. God has given me the wisdom and understanding to hold on to His commandments. I am going to defeat you in Jesus' name because God's Word makes me wiser than you, because greater is He that is in me than he that is in the world." Speak these words out clear and loud when these "can't" words start to come to your mind. Tell them: "I can and surely will have children because God said that 'I can do all things through Christ who gives me strength.'" (Philippians 4: 13)

Scientific background

The dictionary defines infertility as the inability to produce offspring. For a pregnancy to occur a woman must be healthy and be ovulating - that is having her monthly periods, and producing a healthy egg each month. A man must also be producing healthy sperms. Sexual intercourse must also be taking place for one of the millions of sperm ejaculated by the man to travel through the woman's Fallopian tubes and fertilise an egg released from her ovaries. The eggs will fertilise in the Fallopian tube before finally embedding itself in the womb.

Infertility is suggested only if a couple has had unprotected intercourse for one year without a pregnancy. Listed below are some reasons why a pregnancy could fail to occur in the female:

* Damage to the Fallopian tubes or where the tubes have been removed because of congenital defects.

* Hormone problems.

* Ovulation problems, etc.

For the male, problems could arise either in the area of sperm production, or congenital defects etc. It is estimated that about 100 million couples are affected by infertility world-wide. Thirty percent of infertility is due to male factors, thirty per cent to female factors and the remaining forty per cent can be attributed to both partners.

Through the leadership of the Holy Spirit, we are going on a long journey through the pages of the Bible as we deal with each area of male infertility.

First we will see what the symptoms are and then what God has to say about them. We shall be covering areas such as sperm production and congenital problems and much more. God bless you as you read.

Chapter Three

Azoospermia

Azoospermia

This simply describes the absence of sperm from the semen. In this case the man is not producing any sperm at all. Azoospermia may be a disorder present from the time of birth or may develop at a later stage in life. This is one of the main cause of infertility in males.

The Word of God will work for any problem that causes absence of sperm production, in case I did not mention the name of the problem you may be facing.

Congenital azoospermia

This is where the person is born with no ability to produce sperm at all.

Listed below are some of the reasons that can lead to congenital azoospermia.

Klinefeither's Syndrome

This is a chromosome abnormality. This is where a man has an extra or deleted sex chromosome. This leads in turn to increased testosterone (male sex hormone). The normal compliment of sex chromosomes for the male is XY but in this case a man could have XXY making one extra X or he could have XXXY or even more. This disorder leads to development of female features like breast enlargement etc. The body looks feminine rather than male. The testes remain small and the affected male remains infertile due to lack of sperm production. Medically there is no cure because the testes remain a mass of scar tissue and are small in size.

Undescended testes

This is also a problem that a man can be born with. What are testes? Every male child is born with two testes. They are the sex organs that produce sperm and the male sex hormone, testosterone.

This is what happens early in the development of a male foetus; the testes start to form within the abdomen; this is in response to hormones produced by the mother and hormones produced in the testes themselves. The testes gradually start to descend through the inguinal canal in the groin and by the time the baby is born, it has reached the surface of the body where it hangs suspended in a pouch of skin called the scrotum.

However, in some men the testes may have failed to descend properly into the scrotum or may have descended into an abnormal position when the man was a child; they may have gone untreated for so long that they may have stopped producing sperm. Having been kept warm for too long they have lost all their ability to produce sperm.

Absence of the Vas Deferens

This tube is narrow and is on each side of the body. Its main purpose is to carry and store sperm released from the testes and the epididymis. Sperm and seminal fluids are passed through the Vas Deferens into the urethra during ejaculation. Absence of the Vas Deferens could also lead to infertility.

Cystic Fibrosis

This is a genetic disease that affects the lungs and pancreas and may also cause defects of the Vas Deferentia.

Orchitis

This is caused by the mumps virus and may also lead to stoppage of sperm production or it could lower production.

FSH (Follicle Stimulating Hormones)

Where the pituitary gland does not produce enough FSH, (Follicle Stimulating Hormones) which a man needs for sperm production, puberty fails to take place and no sperm or very little is produced by such males.

There are cases where puberty takes place but the man's testes fail to function properly. This could also lead to azoospermia.

Sexually transmitted disease

Gonorrhoea

leads to inflammation of the epididymis and testes which could, if not treated early, leads to blockage of the ducts; this causes infertility.

Syphilis

Is an infectious disease caused by the bacteria *myco-bacterium tuberculosis;* it causes inflammation which could lead to infertility.

Surgery in the groin area

Surgery in the groin area is usually performed to repair a hernia or lower a boy's undescended testes; it could in many cases lead to stoppage of sperm production.

Medication

Most of the commonly used medicinal drugs may interfere with sperm production.

Certain anti-cancer drugs destroy the ability of the testes to produce sperm. High dose x-ray for cancer therapy could affect sperm production. Anti-depressants (doxepin, imigramine) may cause testicular swelling.

Sterilisation operation

This is a very serious decision for any man to take. In this case the Vas Deferentia, the tubes the sperm travels through are cut. After the operation, the man continues to ejaculate as normal, but the semen no longer carries sperm, which are now reabsorbed within the testes. A lot of men, after this operation, may find that their circumstances change and they remarry and desire to have more children but, since they have been sterilised, this becomes impossible. Many try to have the operation reversed and are successful but there are those who are not. With Christ it is possible.

Torsion of the testes

This is where due to the testes being unusually mobile within the scrotum, the spermatic cord becomes twisted, leading to severe pain and swelling of the testes. If this condition is not treated within a few hours, it could lead to permanent damage of the testes and sperm production could cease.

What the Bible offers

For those men who have been told by their specialist they are not producing any sperm, I want to introduce you to Jesus Christ today. He has the answers in the Bible (His Word) for the solution of all sperm production problems.

Under the clear guidance of the Holy Spirit, we are going to take a journey into the Word of God, the Bible, to find out all God has to say through His Son, Jesus Christ, to all the men who face this problem. The Bible says "the Lord led us through the barren wilderness, through a land of deserts and rifts, a land of drought and darkness, a land where no one lives. I brought you into a fertile land to eat its fruits and rich produce." (Jeremiah 2 : 6-7) Maybe today you are walking in a land, where there is drought, and darkness, and you are saying that there is no way out of this land of pain. I want to point you to my Lord Jesus Christ and let you know that if you will come to Him, He will lead you out to a fertile land, where you will have all the children you want.

Hagar (Genesis 21 :14-17)

The first person we will meet is a woman. God indeed has a sense of humour; this woman faced a problem like yours. Here we see God using a woman to solve a man's sperm production problem. The best specialist in the world may have told you there is no way again for you to produce sperm but the Bible says: "God split the rocks in the desert and gave them water as abundant as the seas; he brought streams out of a rocky cliff and made waters flow down like rivers." (Psalms 78: 15-16)

How many times have you seen a rock and expected that water will flow out of it? But the Bible says that when God split that rock, the water flowed like a sea. No matter how dry your testes are God is able to do the same for you, for nothing is too hard for the Lord.

Now we continue on our journey to meet this lady. Her name was Hagar - she was Abraham's mistress. One day, he sent her away after she had a baby boy for him. It reads like this:

> Early the next morning, Abraham took some food and a skin of water and gave them to Hagar. He set them on her shoulder and then sent her off with the boy. She went on her

way and wandered in the desert of Beersheba. When the water in the skin was gone, she put the boy under one of the bushes, then she went off and sat nearby, about a bow-shot away, for she thought, "I cannot watch the boy die." As she sat there nearby she began to sob. God heard the boy crying and the angel of God called to Hagar from heaven and said to her, "What is the matter, Hagar? Do not be afraid. God has heard the boy crying as he lies there." (Genesis 21: 14-17)

Then God opened her eyes and she saw a well of water, so she went and filled the skin with water and gave the boy a drink. (Genesis 21: 19)

"God heard the boy crying" was the statement made by the Angel of God? The boy Ishmael was the son of a slave woman, the offspring of a failure of faith. They mocked Isaac and were sent away into a desert with only one skin of water between mother and son. What is a desert? A desert is described as a desolate region, a dry barren region incapable of supporting much life.

These two found themselves in a place incapable of supporting life - you also find yourself being told that you are incapable of producing life. This situation is the same, and the same principle that God used here He will also use to bring deliverance to you. When Hagar was sent away she passed out of the sight of Abraham and his family but not out of the sight of God; nor were they beyond his care or government.

When Abraham sent her away, God was still with her and guiding her and protecting her and her son. For He is the God who has given us His Word: "I will never leave you or forsake you." Abraham did not need her anymore, but the God who created her was with her, watching over her and protecting her on her journey.

"God opened her eyes and she saw a well of water." God provided water for them to preserve their life.

Some of you wonderful men of God may well be saying in your heart, "This doctor's report is so bad, it is over for me. I can never be a biological father during my lifetime." Be of good cheer. I want to encourage you today; Jesus has not changed. He is the same yesterday, today and forever. He can and will help you if you will dare to call upon Him and trust Him. God sees you crying and He has heard all your cries. He has seen all your pain and He sends you His word to heal you.

This is what Hagar said about God: "I have now seen the one who sees me." (Genesis 16: 13) God sees you even when you think He doesn't. He sees your pain even when you think He doesn't. He desires to bless you even when you think He doesn't.

God sees you

Even if the best specialists in the world have told you that you cannot produce sperm ever again in your life - no matter the reason you have been given, no matter how bad the medical report - you can boldly say, "The God who made streams to flow in a desert, the God who made a well of water for Hagar in the desert is more than able to make me produce life. He is able to revive and repair any damage that I cannot see, because He alone is the God who sees me."

Hagar thought they would die in that desert but God had seen her. You may say to yourself, "There is no hope of my ever being a father," but the Bible says, "All things are possible to those who believe." (Matthew 17: 20) The Bible also says: "The desert and the parched land will be glad; the wilderness will rejoice and blossom. Like the crocus, it will burst into bloom; it will rejoice greatly and shout for joy." (Isaiah 35: 1-2) In this scripture the Bible talks of wilderness and parched pasture land. Here it is talking of the condition which can only be described as parched, that is, affording no pasturage.

The Bible affirms that the parched pasture land, "shall be glad." God promises in His Word that even though the best doctors in the world might have told you that your testes "are parched - no sperm", God is saying, "No! No!" Those testes will break forth, will burgeon, will blossom and bear much fruit (children) to the glory of God. Then God concludes by saying to you, His beloved son, that you will greatly rejoice and shout for joy. I want to encourage you. Reach out and receive His blessing like a little baby; don't doubt but only believe.

If you will believe, very soon you will be a father. Your home will be full of beautiful children, because the Lord is able; not only is He able but is eager to bless you.

The second Bible account I want us to look at is found in the book of Numbers.

Aaron's rod sprouts (Numbers 17: 5)

The children of Israel grumbled so much about Moses and Aaron. One day God decided to stop all these by indicating powerfully who He had chosen. He told all the elders of the Israelites to present their staffs in the tent of meeting. "The staff belonging to the man I choose will sprout." (Numbers 17: 5) "Moses placed the staffs before the Lord in the tent of testimony. The next day Moses entered the tent of testimony and saw that Aaron's staff which represented the house of Levi, had not only sprouted but had budded and blossomed and produced almonds." (Numbers 17: 7-8)

What is a staff? It is a stick carried in the hand for use in walking or as a weapon; a supporting rod.

What is a bud? - a plant puts forth buds to develop by way of outgrowth so as to reproduce asexually by forming and developing buds.

Blossom: This is the flower of a plant, especially the flower that produces edible fruits - the mass of bloom on a single plant, a high point or stage of development.

Almonds: the edible oval nut of a small tree of the rose family.

What am I saying here? A dead piece of wood and the power of God. I have described what happened to that rod or staff from the time it was put into the house of God. Here we see a dead piece of wood, taken into the house of God and within twenty-four hours it had budded, blossomed and had borne almond nuts - can you imagine that? This rod had no life force; it was not planted, yet it budded at God's command. Imagine what God can do for you if you choose to come to Jesus Christ, for you will become a man with the blood and life of God flowing through you. God is able in an instant to get everything working in perfect order for you. If God can do this for a rod (piece of dead wood) because He wanted to show His approval for the owner of that rod, then there is no reason why He cannot make your testes produce sperm again. God is more than able. For the Bible says, "In Christ we will bear much fruit." (John 15: 5). Our third Bible account is in the book of Luke 5.

We have toiled all night in vain

Our Lord Jesus Christ is full of mercy and compassion and His Word has not changed. His Word is just as powerful today as it was when he spoke it forth thousands of years ago. His Word is pregnant with the very life of God. He said "the words that I speak to you they are spirit and life."(John 6: 63). His word is still powerful and relevant for our every need today just as it was thousands of years ago.

"One day as Jesus was standing by the lake of Gennesaret....

He saw at the water's edge two boats, left there by the fishermen, who were washing their nets. He got into one of the boats, the one belonging to Simon, and asked him to put out a little from the shore. Then he sat down and taught the people from the boat. When he had finished speaking, he said to Simon, "put out into deep water, and let down the nets for a catch." Simon answered "master we have worked hard all night and haven't caught anything. But because you say so, I will let down the nets."
When they had done so, they caught such a large number of fish that their nets began to break. So they signaled to their partner in the other boat to come and help them, and they came and filled both boats so full that they began to sink. When Simon Peter saw this, he fell at Jesus knees and said, "go away from me, Lord; I am a sinful man." For he and his companions were astonished at the catch of fish they had taken. (Luke 5:2-9).

In this miracle we once again see the incredible acts of our lord Jesus. Jesus met the disciples at the edge of the water. They were washing their nets after toiling all night in vain to catch fish to maintain their family and their livelihood, these men were professional fishermen; but on this ocasssion they had toiled all night in vain. What is to toil? The dictionary says - it is to labour with pain and fatigue of body or mind, to move or make progress painfully or laboriously. Hard and unremitting work.

May be today you are feeling like this men, you have toiled all night in vain. You have done all you can to get your wife pregnant and nothing has happened. You are tired of all the sperm count business, you are fade up with the ups and down and like the disciples you are busy washing your net and waiting for a turn around. I want to ecourage you that the same Jesus who came to these fishermen has come to you and from today your story must change.

Our Lord Jesus in his usual way came to them at the water edge and told them to "put out into deep water, and let down their nets for a catch." Simon Peter answered, "master we have worked hard all night and haven't caught anything. But because you say so, I will let down the nets." Jesus has come to you through this book you are reading and is asking you to let down your nets for a catch. Today I want to ask you a question; have you toiled all night in vain?

Have you done all you know to do and that pregnancy does not seem to be coming forth? Now it is time to hand the whole situation to Jesus Christ. The One who blessed Simon Peter and his partners with more fish in one day, than they had caught in a whole year can do the same for you. Azoospermia is nothing to the Lord. All you need to hear is one word from the Master and the storm you are facing becomes still and calm. I want to tell you that Jesus loves you and azoospermia will no longer torment you after today. Today is the day to enter into Gods rest and tell him to take control of your net. Today is the day you say to the Lord, "show me where the catch is, I am ready to obey your word, I am ready to let down my net for a catch because you say so. Help me Lord!"

No matter what you been told or what you've been through; the Master is able to make it right for you have. The One who did it for the tired fishermen is telling you today, I am able. Take your rest in Him and through faith believe that He is able to bless you with all the children you need. It is now time to fill your home with the joy of children. As you start to praise God, and walk in obedience to His Word your life will be perfected by his Word and the glory that comes in obedience to his word.

What if Simon Peter had refused to cast his nets for a catch when the Lord told him to do so? He was tired but he obeyed the Lord and experienced a mighty breakthrough. Most of the time our circumstances may want to hinder us from obeying the Lord but If you will act by faith today you will experience the same mighty breakthrough these third men experienced when they obeyed the Lord. Why not? Our Lord is no respecter of persons. If he did it for them he can also do it for you.

The Bible also says that nothing shall separate us from the love of Christ. A sperm production problem is not something which should separate you from the love of God. Just hand this so-called problem to God and see what God will do with it. The Bible says God works everything together for the good of those who love Him.

Remember, God shows no favouritism, (Romans 2: 11) and God never changes. What He did for someone else, if you can find it in His Word, He will do it for you. He is faithful.

I have used these Bible accounts to encourage you and let you know that God is able and faithful. First we see God intervene in a desert to provide water for Hagar to preserve her life and that of her son. Then we see God giving life to a piece of dead wood to show His support was for the owner of that staff. We then see the Lord intervene in the life of third men to bless the work of their hands. Just imagine what God can do for you, as a man saved with the blood of Jesus Christ. I can guarantee you great victories await you, if you say yes to God. If you are already a child of God, you may have gone through the Bible and not really understood or found the solution to the problem you are facing and you may have given up. God wants you to take what has been written down and come to Him by faith and receive your inheritance. "Sons are a heritage from the Lord, children a reward from him." (Psalms 127: 3) If you really come to God and believe in Him and His Word, then before you know it that beautiful wife of yours will be pregnant. Why not? - he has promised us in his Word. No good thing will be withheld from those who walk uprightly.

Points of action

- ❖ Come to God through Jesus Christ by faith.
- ❖ Tell God about all areas of the medical report you have received.
- ❖ Do whatever God tells you to do.
- ❖ Believe He has blessed you as you have asked Him.
- ❖ Confess your blessing from your mouth.
- ❖ Start to praise Him by faith, thanking Him for His faithfulness.

Now make a -:

Confession

Father, in the name of Jesus, I bless you and I thank you that I am a man redeemed with the blood of Jesus Christ. I am above and not under, I am blessed and highly favoured. God is on my side. The Word of God helps me, I am a winner. Iam free from the curse of the law. The blessings of Abraham is mine. I am a father of many children. Azoospermia is far from me; my testes are producing sperm normally because the Word of God is active, it has quickly and actively put my testes in working order; my testes are making sperm normally in the way God intended them to. The Holy Spirit of God regenerates, I thank God that His Word imparts fresh life to every organ in my body, my testes are in perfect working order; Anything that is missing or damaged inside my body is being recreated and brought back into existence by His Word. I am a father of many children in the name of Jesus.

Chapter Four

Oligospermia

Oligospermia simply means that a man is producing very few sperm. A man will normally produce more than twenty million sperm per millilitre of semen to stand a good chance of impregnating his wife, but in most cases of oligospermia he will find himself producing very little sperm. Oligospermia may be temporary or permanent. These are some of the medical reasons given for this.

- smoking
- inflammation of the testes
- alcohol abuse
- treatment with certain drugs
- over-tiredness due to overwork (This also tends to reduce sperm count.)

Over-heated testes

A man's testes need to be kept cool for optimum sperm production; too many warm baths, or being over-weight can reduce sperm production, in the latter case because the testes are constantly clasped between the fat of the man's thighs, thus increasing the temperature of the testes by keeping them warmer than normal. Tight underwear and trousers can also increase the heat of the testes hindering them from working effectively, and leading to low sperm production.

Varicoceles

These are veins surrounding the testes. This condition affects a man's left testis exclusively. The condition is thought to impede fertility by allowing increased heat in the affected testis. Spermicidal metabolic toxins may build up as a result of lack of drainage in the affected vein; because of this there is inadequate circulation in the testicles thereby leading to low sperm count.

What the Bible offers

In the Name of Jesus Christ, the name that is above every name, I bring you the good news that Jesus Christ is Lord. I want every man who has been diagnosed with a low sperm count to meet Jesus Christ for yourself today. Travelling through the pages of the Bible with you under the guidance of the Holy Spirit we will deal with the problem of low sperm count. You will be amazed to discover that the Bible stories you may or may not have known hold the key to the solution of your problem.

Jesus and the multitude (John 6: 5-13)

Jesus was preaching to a multitude of people and they followed Him because they saw the miraculous signs that He had performed on the sick. (John 6: 2) When Jesus looked up and saw a great crowd coming toward Him, He said to Philip, "Where shall we buy bread for these people to eat?" He asked this only to test him, for Jesus already had in mind what He was going to do. Philip answered him, "Eight months' wages would not buy enough bread for each one to have a bite!" Another of His disciples, Andrew, Simon Peter's brother, spoke up: "Here is a boy with five small barley loaves and two small fish, but how far will they go among so many?"

Our Lord moves

Jesus said, "Make the people sit down." There was plenty of grass in that place and the men sat down, about five thousand of them. Jesus then took the loaves, gave thanks and distributed to those who were seated as much as they wanted. He did the same with the fish.

When they had all had enough to eat, He said to His disciples, "Gather the pieces of barley loaves that are left over by those who have eaten." (John 6: 5-13) "So they gathered and filled twelve baskets with the leftovers from the five barley loaves." (John 6: 13)

For any man facing low sperm production, I invite you to follow me through this journey carefully as the Holy Spirit brings light into this issue of low sperm production. "How can I have enough sperm to impregnate my wife?" *"Where shall we buy bread for these people to eat?"* Jesus put a great problem before His disciples. You face a great problem today. Our Lord's eyes were forever going to and fro throughout the whole world. He always saw before anyone else did and He saw differently from all others. On this occasion He saw the weary, fainting, hungry crowd of people, five thousand in all. The Lord knew all men; He knew how far they had travelled and He knew they were hungry and tired, and He knew what they needed and He also knew that He could supply all their needs. Today, Jesus is able and He will also supply you with all the sperm you need; He also sees all your pains and will bring joy to you.

Man's impossibilities

The difficulty and impossibility of a solution to this question is revealed in the answer of Philip and Andrew. Philip calculated the cost; Andrew emphasised the inadequacy of their resources. All they saw were impossibilities.

Today, you may face the same impossibilities; the doctors may have told you, "No way - your sperm count is too low; you can't father children, etc." Please follow carefully as we continue on this adventure.

Andrew now came up with a venture of faith. "Here is a boy with five barley loaves and two fishes." He then casually makes a remark of amusement. "But how far can these go among so many?" He laughed at his own suggestion. It sounded stupid to him - he could not see a solution - and it seemed totally impossible for him to perceive how these people could be fed that day. Common-sense is not always equal in measure to Christ's presence and power. He satisfies the thirsty soul, feeds the hungry with His own supply, and heals the inner body.

Our Lord moves into action

Jesus moved into action. Jesus said, "Make the people sit down." He took the loaves, gave thanks and distributed to those who were seated and they ate as much as they wanted. He did the same with the fish. When they had eaten enough, He said to His disciples, "Gather the left-overs." So they gathered them and filled twelve baskets with the five barley loaves left over by those who had eaten. (John 6: 10-13)

If you have been told you are not producing enough sperm to impregnate your wife today, I want you to know something - what you need to know is that Jesus Christ is the one who knows what to do. He who took five loaves and two fishes and fed five thousand, is able to use just one sperm from your body to produce a child for you - no hassles. Please note that, after the bread had fed five thousand, they had twelve baskets left over. Well, you are producing more than enough. If you have more than seven sperm - you have a surplus in Jesus' name. With Christ, a hopeless scarcity becomes abundant, exceeding what is required. He supplies abundantly if only permitted. This is the principle of divine performance. This is the sign of the supernatural - superabundance of divine provision. Low sperm count is nothing to the Lord. He can right it for you without any sweat, if you will dare to believe Him.

The second journey I would like us to take is through the book of I Samuel to prove to you once and for all that little is much when God is in it. Low sperm production cannot stop you from having children if you call on Jesus.

David and Goliath

This is the story of David and Goliath. Goliath was a Philistine giant, a mighty soldier. One day, he decided to start tormenting God's people. In one statement, this is what he said. "'I defy the ranks of Israel! Give me a man and let us fight each other.' On hearing the Philistine's words, Saul and all Israel were dismayed and terrified." (1 Samuel 17: 10-11)

He kept on at them every day and, while all this was going on, David was sent to the camp to bring provision to his older brothers. While there, David overheard all these threats this Philistine soldier was hurling at God's people. David said to Saul, the King of Israel: "Let no one lose heart on account of this Philistine; your servant will go and fight him." I also want to encourage you that low sperm production may have tormented you, but God is able to give you victory; do not lose heart. Saul replied, "You are not able to go out against this Philistine and fight him - you are only a boy and he has been fighting from his youth." (I Samuel 17: 32-33)

Please don't listen to anyone who wants to justify why you cannot produce enough sperm or why you can't father children. Listen carefully to what David did, and said, and apply this truth to yourself and before you know it, your beautiful wife will be pregnant in Jesus' name.

While the king was telling David it was not possible, David told him how he had killed lions and bears with his bare hands when those animals turned on him. Today, you can, in the name of Jesus, turn around low sperm count and totally prevent it from being a problem in your life. Through Jesus Christ you can walk away smiling at low sperm count as God gives you an effortless victory. If you will dare to believe God and His written Word, your victory is just around the corner. Turn around that corner and it is there waiting for you. Why not? Jesus is the master of the storm. He is the one fighting the battle. It is not you. The battle belongs to the Lord.

Confidence in the Lord

David then made this statement to show where his boasting came from: "The Lord who delivered me from the paws of the lion and the paws of the bear will deliver me from the hand of this Philistine." (I Samuel 17: 37)

If you are not afraid to take your stand and declare the Word of God, then the same God who delivered David from the paws of the lion and bear will also deliver you from infertility, in Jesus' name.

One is enough

Then David "chose five smooth stones from the stream and put them in the pouch of his shepherd's bag and, with his sling in his hand, he approached the Philistine." (I Samuel 17: 40)

When the Philistine came closer and saw that David was but a boy, he despised him. He said to David. "Am I a dog that you come to me with sticks?" A lot of people will want to mock you, especially if you are a Christian and cannot father children because of low sperm production - they will ridicule you and make you feel you are a loser for serving or trusting God.

Please note what David said to the Philistine: "You come against me with a sword, spear and javelin, but I come against you in the name of the Lord almighty, the God of the armies of Israel, whom you have defied." This is exactly what infertility does to people - it tries to defy you. It comes in the disguise of low sperm production, It comes in disguise of one thing or the other but it is an enemy - it is not a friend.

Victory with one stone

As the Philistine moved closer to attack him, David ran quickly towards the battle line to meet him. Reaching into his bag and taking out a stone, he slung it and struck the Philistine on his forehead. The stone sank into his forehead and he fell face down on the ground. So David triumphed over the Philistine with a sling and a stone; without a sword in his hand, he struck down the Philistine and killed him.

David said these words: "The battle belongs to the Lord." (I Samuel 17: 47) If a man produces ten million sperm cells a day in his testes, the doctors say he needs to be producing about twenty million sperm per hpf (60-80 million total sperm in 4 CCs) to impregnate his wife. So, if a man is producing four million sperm per one hpf in 4 CCs), it is said to be low. During love-making, a man ejaculates about 500-800 million sperm into the vagina; each of the sperm released is capable of fertilising an ovum. But as they travel upwards (propelled by their whip-like tails) more than half are killed by acidic vagina secretions. Many more die during the journey up through the cervix and into the Fallopian tubes; the journey can take from one to six hours and in the end only one sperm wins the race.

Fertilisation

As the sperm swims towards the mature ovum in the Fallopian tube, fertilisation takes place when *one* of the sperms penetrates the mature ovum. Once one penetrates, the egg closes itself up and no more sperm is allowed into the ovum; thus only one sperm can win the race. After penetration, the nuclei (which contain the genetic material) of the sperm and ovum fuse and the body and tail of the sperm drop off. At the end of all this vast sperm production, only one sperm is needed to create new life. Here a man is producing four million and it is said to be a low count, when all he really needs is "one".

All you need is one sperm

David chose five stones but all he needed to accomplish his task and hit his target was one stone. All you need today to impregnate and create new life, to hit your target, is one sperm, not even two. If, like David, you can say, "The battle belongs to the Lord; I may be producing very low sperm count, but I have more than one and one is all that is really needed," then, just as David killed Goliath, you can confidently run home to your wife and say: "Darling, we don't need even five sperm per hpf in Jesus' name; all we need is one and I have that one because this battle has now been handed over to the Lord. "

I now want to link both Bible accounts together to encourage you and let you know that little is much when God is there.

Jesus already knew what He would do before He asked the disciples for a suggestion. David already knew that with God's help he was able to kill that giant. He also estimated that with five stones he could accomplish this, but because God was fighting the battle, all he needed was one stone. When Jesus is at hand, everything that is missing or needed is always made available. In His presence there can never be any lack.

Jesus always sees any impending danger and difficulty. He knows the complications that the circumstances are likely to create and He knows the best way out. You may be wondering about the complications involved in whatever God may ask you to do, but He has already taken care of it; if you dare to trust Him, He Himself knows what to do.

I want to leave you with this advice. You don't need to be producing 60-80 million sperm per 4 CCs, all you need to be producing is *one,* in Christ, to be able to father a child. All you need is Jesus Christ and don't even pretend you can better the suggestion of his disciples on that day He fed the five thousand with two fishes and five loaves; but you can come boldly to Him, bring the report of the low sperm count which the doctors have given you, and present it to the Lord; then you can be confident in your heart that whatever God has in mind to do, He is able to do it with your resources. I know not but you know, Lord; I trust You and all I ask is that I be directed by Your wisdom so that I shall be enabled by Your power to succeed in Jesus' name. Just as you led David to triumph over a giant with one stone and a sling, so also you will lead me with the one anointed sperm to fertilise an egg and create a baby in Jesus' name.

I have taken the time to read and study materials from fertility clinics and read many books on this issue. Many fertility doctors of our day have no better advice than the disciples of Jesus in His day - *"Send them away that they may buy for themselves bread."* But the fainting, helpless condition of the multitudes demanded that a miracle be worked.

There is much lack and much thirst in our times. We live in a day of mighty famine; man in so many instances is being offered only the husks that belong to the swine.

In recognition of this helpless, pitiful condition, God is now bringing a banquet of abundant supply; men will appreciate God's wonderful provision in every area of life as they behold His unquenchable desire to fill all men with all they need to multiply. 100 million couples worldwide are estimated to face this problem. Thus you can clearly see that what we need is not the inadequacy of our own scientific researches, and the inability of our own power, but the power to see God's abilities and believe that He is able to meet the needs of all men at all times, as we behold His power and glory. As we acknowledge the one who used five small barley loaves and two small fishes to feed five thousand people and still collected twelve baskets of left-overs; the left-overs were still more than what He started out with initially. The one who fought David's battle with Goliath, who used one stone to triumph over the giant Goliath is the one you need to see today. As you stare into his face defeat flees from your life and your life becomes a life of victory.

Talk to Him and let Him talk back to you. Believe Him and let Him bless you. Why not? His greatest desire is to bless you. Below are some points of action to help you - go to Him any way you know; if you are sincere He will surely meet with you and I can guarantee you your life will never be the same again.

Points of action

❖ Come to God through faith.
❖ Tell God about all your medical reports.
❖ Tell Him what you would like Him to do for you.
❖ Condemn every negative report.
❖ Declare your victory in Jesus' name.
❖ Start to praise God for His goodness and mercy.

Make a confession

Father, in the name of Jesus, I bless you. I thank you that I am a man that is redeemed with the blood of Jesus Christ. I am above and not under, I am blessed and highly favoured. Low sperm count is far from me. I expose my testes to the Word of God and declare in the name of Jesus, that my testes are working normally. I subject my testes to the Word of God, which is effective, and I declare that my testes are producing enough sperm in the way that God designed them to work. In the name of Jesus. God looks on me with favour and makes me fruitful and increases my numbers. He keeps his covenant with me. While my wife is still recovering from last year's childbirth, it is time to make room for even more babies. God loves me. He walks with me. He has destroyed the yoke and bars of low sperm count and has enabled me to become a father of healthy children with my head held high. (Leviticus 26:3-13). The Father is rebuilding the old waste-places of my life, I'm like a green pine tree; my fruitfulness comes from the Father.(Hosea 14:8) All that the canker worm have eaten the Father is now restoring to me. I love You Father in Jesus name-Amen.

Chapter Five

Impotence

A man can be said to be impotent if he is unable to achieve or maintain an erection. This is the most distressing and embarrassing thing that can happen to a man's self esteem. The most common causes of impotence are psychological factors which may be temporary, e.g. fatigue, stress, anxiety, or guilt that might originate from some childhood experience. Other factors include diabetes mellitus, or a disorder of the endocrine system, or even damage to the spinal cord; alcohol abuse could lead to impotence. Drugs like anti-depressants, anti-psychotic drugs, hypertensive drugs and diuretic drugs could all cause impotence.

Premature ejaculation

This is one of the most common sexual problems men face, especially in adolescence. Premature ejaculation occurs when a man ejaculates before or very soon after penetration. In most cases this could be the result of over-stimulation or anxiety over sexual performance and there could even be an underlying cause where it becomes frequent.

A lot of men have penile implants inserted in the penis to help them with the problem of impotence. Where impotence is caused by a disease, it is said to be permanent.

Silicon splint

This is inserted in the tissue of the upper surface of the penis. When this is done, the penis can be inserted in the vagina but will not increase in size.

Inflatable prosthesis

Here an inflatable prosthesis is inserted into the penis. This will make the penis larger and firmer for intercourse and is operated by squeezing a small bulb placed into the scrotum.

What the Bible offers (John 5: 1-8)

In the name of Jesus Christ, I invite you to take a journey with me through the pages of the Bible under the leadership of the Holy Spirit to see what the Word of God has to tell us about impotence. Our Lord Jesus Christ made this statement. "For just as the Father raises the dead and gives them life, even so the Son will give life to whom he is pleased to give it." (John 5: 21)

I want us to get one thing clear from here on; Jesus is the giver of life. He alone can give life, He alone gives life. Wherever there is death, Jesus brings abundant life. We will now take a journey through the Bible to see how Jesus dealt with impotence, to learn from it as well and apply it to your case.

Jesus at a hospital

> Some time later, Jesus went up to Jerusalem for a feast of the Jews. Now there is in Jerusalem near the Sheep Gate a pool, which in Aramaic is called Bethesda and which is surrounded by five covered colonnades. Here a great number of disabled people used to lie - the blind, the lame the paralysed. One who was there had been an invalid for thirty-eight years. When Jesus saw him lying there and learned that he had been in this condition for a long time, he asked him, "Do you want to get well?"
>
> "Sir," the invalid replied, "I have no one to help me into the pool when the water is stirred. While I am trying to get in, someone else goes down ahead of me."
>
> Then Jesus said to him, "Get up! Pick up your mat and walk." At once the man was cured; he picked up his mat and walked. (John 5: 1-8)

Here we see Jesus in a hospital of that time. One of the greatest things that strikes me about our Lord is that wherever suffering or misery exists, there He will always be found, changing lives and bringing hope.

Bethesda (which means house of mercy or house of compassion) was a place where suffering and misery walked hand in hand. Many people once given up by doctors were told then, as now, things like "there is no hope", "we can do no more for you". Here they were all gathered, hoping and waiting for a miracle, but nothing happened for this old man for thirty-eight years.

What is impotence?

Impotence is a weakness affecting or reducing the strength or vigour of a part of the body - here in this man's case it was his limbs. In your case, it may be your penis, but, in all situations, Jesus is able. Even those men with penile implants who have been told their impotence is permanent, need to get this message clear in their spirit. Nothing in life is permanent; God's Word always overrules every impossibility man faces. God's Word is final and every situation we face is subject to obey God's Word.

It is not over, until it's over

After thirty-eight years, this man thought it was over but as my pastor would say, "It is not over until it's over." Jesus is the physician who not only understands the case but has all the ability to deal with it and He definitely delivers. The doctors may have given you the news that nothing more can be done to help you. Your case, like this man's, may seem hopeless but Jesus, the great physician, is more than able to work it out for you.

The will of man

Jesus asked this man one question: "Will you be made whole?" This question sounds needless in this situation. The fact that the man was at the pool is an indication he wanted to be healed, but still the Lord asked him. Why? Because when God created man, He gave man the right to choose. He gave man a will; every man has a will to choose. God will not force you to be healed or even to serve Him; you will have to choose what you want.

The will of man is a gift of God to man and it plays a large part in physical as well as spiritual recovery. Our Lord never, and will never, do anything for anyone against their will. Statements made by our Lord like, "If any man wills, let him come unto me and drink; if any man will open the door, I will come onto him and sup with him and he with me," indicate this is so. Man's consent is the first step towards divine blessing. Christ is willing to help the helpless anywhere if the helpless are willing to acknowledge their helplessness and reveal a readiness to be healed.

Today, if you desire to part ways with impotence you must be ready to call on Jesus Christ and tell Him what you want. You must be willing to accept personally that what He did for this man He can also do for you; then you are ready to receive from Him total healing from impotence and every other need.

The hopefulness of this question

When our Lord asked this man if he was willing to be healed, this man did not answer directly; he went into a sad tale of how he did not have anyone to help him into the pool, when the water was stirred. Here we see a man in trouble, putting his hope in troubled waters. This man indeed had resigned himself to his fate. Little did he know the one he was speaking to was the resurrection and the life. Little did he know the one who spoke to him was the one who is able to raise all that is dead - be it limbs, penis or dreams. Jesus is the resurrection and the life. In His presence no death can remain.

Our Lord's command

"Rise, take up your bed and walk." This is a most extraordinary prescription. It is a powerful pharmacy which can work that way. To step into the pool seemed wonderful indeed, but this is even more wonderful. "Hey man, you mean I don't have to step into the pool; this is cool, man. You mean I should just get up and walk - just get up and go home." This sounded too good to be true and yet it was all true. His nightmare of thirty-eight years was over. He was whole again. In a twinkle of an eye Jesus Christ stepped in and brought healing to thirty-eight years of misery. What a mighty God we serve.

Use of penile implants is over for you

Penile implants are good and they have helped you but today in Jesus' name, you can be whole again; you can be free from them; your penis will rise again and work in Jesus' name. What He did to the man's limbs He can do for the penis. Here we see the Lord asking the man to do the impossible. His impotent limbs had not held him for thirty-eight years, yet they are commanded to do what they are ordained to do. A palsied man is ordered to walk off with his bed - not only walk but walk and carry his mat with him.

Every human power and medical science had failed to help this man even in the early stages of his impotence; now in the grips of its chronic condition, the sufferer is told to act as if he had never known suffering. The best specialist in the world may have told you that there is no way that your penis will function normally, but learning from what happened in this man's case, you can discover there is total restoration in the name of Jesus, in any situation that is handed over to the Lord. He is able to bring total restoration and quickly too.

Obedience is the key to total victory in every area of life. It leads to great accomplishment; it brings break-through. Immediately our Lord said to this man, "Rise up, take your bed and walk," he immediately did it. This time he did not have time to start saying, "Why? This is not possible." He quickly obeyed without thinking, forgetting that those limbs had been impotent for thirty-eight years. He did not even have time to say, "Oh! Please, sir, give me a hand," since he did not know who Jesus was; yet something in him told him this was his day. He simply did what he had never done before. As Mike Murdock would say, "If you want God to do something He has never done for you before, He will also be asking you to do what you have never done before." You saw how the man moved when Jesus told him, to get up and walk; as you read this man's life story and faith is released in your heart, God will give you specific instructions. You will know when He does; it will be something you never thought you could do, but as you obey and do it, your victory will be sealed and you will be made whole. Why not? He who did it for the impotent man will do it for you if you will dare to ask Him and believe Him through faith. The Bible says our God shows no favouritism. (Romans 2: 11) Whatever He did for someone else, He will do for you, if you can find it in His Word.

Finally, I bring you the very first scripture the Lord showed me about impotence back in 1994. With the help of this scripture a friend whose husband who was impotent was healed and nine months and one week to the day that I prayed with her, she was holding a beautiful baby boy, to the glory of God.

The Bible says that God commanded man to multiply and increase. "God blessed them and said to them, be fruitful and increase in number, fill the earth and subdue it." (Genesis 1: 28) Not long after this command, the Bible again tells us: "Adam knew his wife (had intercourse with his wife) and she bore Cain." How can a man multiply if he is impotent. You must reject impotence in your life, in Jesus' name.

God told the woman in Genesis 3: 16, "Your desire will be for your husband." What is desire? It means to long or hope for, to express a wish, to wish to have a sexual relationship with your husband. Every woman's desire is for her husband. What is a woman with desire to do with an impotent man? You can clearly see that impotence contradicts God's command in your life. If, as a husband, you are unable to meet the sexual desires of your wife, it means you both have been robbed of God's blessing in your life. The woman's longing is not being met because of impotence.

The Word of God says to us, "Do not deprive each other except by mutual consent, and for a time, so that you may devote yourselves to prayer." (I Corinthians 7: 5) From this scripture you can see that the only permission God has given to abstain from marital conjugation is prayer; beyond that nothing else should be allowed to interfere with this duty. Based on this scripture and the others, this is what I advise you to do.

Points of action

- Reject impotence in Jesus' name.
- Command it to leave your home forever
- Tell God you want to resume a normal relationship with your wife based upon His Word.
- God may ask you to take a step of faith; do whatever He tells you to do.
- Start thanking and praising God by faith. God bless you.
  Now make a confession:

Father, in the name of Jesus, I bless you and worship you. Father, the Bible says that your Word is alive; I take your Word which is alive and speak life back into my penis in the name of Jesus Christ. I am a man that is full of the strength of the Lord. I am a strong man. I have the power and strength of God's divine nature flowing through my body. I am empowered by the living Word of God to live above the natural circumstances of life. I am quickened in my mortal body, the Spirit of the living God quickens my penis. He restores life to every dead organ in my body, He stimulates, rouses, rekindles every part of my reproductive organs that needs these treatments. The powerful Word of God moves fast and accelerates every work that the Word of God is doing in my body. I thank you that all my reproductive organs are working perfectly, because your resurrection power flows in my body through the power of your name. I thank you Father in Jesus' name, Amen.

Chapter Six

Congenital Problems

A congenital disorder simply means an abnormality that is present from birth. It may have been inherited or may have occurred as a result of damage or even an infection in the womb. It may have occurred during the time of birth. Not all congenital disorders are inherited.

During my research for this book, I noticed that some of the congenital disorders led to lack of sperm production.

Listed below are some of the congenital disorders that affect the male reproduction system. In case I do not mention the name of the problem your are facing, don't worry; if it is a congenital problem leading to low sperm or no sperm production, you can take the Word of God relating to these conditions and apply it; and you will receive your miracle in Jesus' name. If the problem is one requiring a creative miracle, then stay here and use the Word to receive your miracle in Jesus' name.

Klinefelter's Syndrome

This is a chromosome abnormality where an extra or deleted chromosome may cause infertility. The problem here is that because of the chromosome abnormalities, a man with this ailment starts to grow feminine features like breasts, etc. The affected male remains infertile because of lack of sperm production. The testes remain small and are just a mass of scar tissue.

Varicoceles

As previously mentioned, these are the veins surrounding the testes; this condition affects almost exclusively the left testis. This is thought to impede fertility by allowing increased heat in the affected testis. This is the result of inadequate circulation through the testicles and this leads to low sperm count in most men.

Abnormal urethral opening

The urethras are the tubes that carry urine from the kidneys to the bladder. They enter the back of the bladder at an angle. In men, the urethra is much longer than in women; it is surrounded by the prostate gland at its upper end and forms a channel through the length of the penis. Any disorders in the male urethra can be very serious. The congenital anomalies like abnormal urethra openings (too high or low on the penis) may contribute to infertility by not allowing the sperm to enter the vagina. If the opening to the penis is incorrect, the semen merely exits the penis outside the vagina.

Absence or blockage of the Vas Deferens

The Vas Deferens is a narrow tube on each side of the body that carries the sperm; it is the sperm tube. It carries and steers the sperm from the testes. A man may have either an absence of or blockage of the Vas Deferens and be unable to transport sperm from the testicles to the urethra. The absence of a Vas Deferens might be the result of a birth defect or injury. The blockage might result in a collection of sperm called a spermatocele. This often becomes a mass in the testicles.

Congenital problems that affect the testes

Every male child is born with two testes and they are the sex organs that produce sperm and the male sex hormone, testosterone.

Early in the development of a male foetus, the testis start to form within the abdomen near his kidney as a response to hormones produced by the mother and hormones produced in the testis of that baby itself. The testis gradually starts to descend through the inguinal canal in the groin and by the time the baby is born it has reached the surface of the body where it hangs suspended in a pouch of skin called the scrotum.

Undescended Testes

However, in most cases the testes may have failed to descend properly into the scrotum or may have descended into an abnormal position when that child was in the womb; if this condition is not treated, it becomes a problem because the testes, having been kept so warm, lose all ability to produce sperm; thus this then leads to infertility.

Ectopic Testes

This is where the testes are absent from the scrotum because they have descended into an abnormal position, either in the groin or the base of the penis. This will normally be discovered after the birth of a male child during a routine physical examination. If the condition is not discovered and treated early it could lead to infertility.

Hypospadias

This is a congenital defect where the penile opening of the urethra is situated on the underside of the penis. The urethral opening may be on the glans (head) or the penis-shaft. In other cases the penis may curve downwards.

Testicular Feminisation Syndrome

This is a rare inherited condition where a person may have all the external appearance of a female, but the affected individual is genetically a male with internal testes. This is a form of intersex. The cause of this syndrome is a defective response of the body's tissue to the male sex hormone, testosterone, even though a normal level of the male hormone is produced. Affected individuals appear to be girls throughout their childhood. At puberty they develop normal female secondary sexual characteristics but menstruation does not occur because there is no uterus and the vagina is short and has a blind ending.

This condition is normally detected at puberty if a girl is found to have an inguinal hernia or swelling in her labia that turn out to be a testis. Otherwise the diagnosis is usually made at puberty, when investigation is carried out to find out why menstruation has not started. A chromosome analysis will be carried out, which will then reveal the girl to have normal male chromosomal status while a blood test will indicate male levels of testosterone (the male sex hormone).

Doctors will normally operate to remove the testes because of the risk of testicular cancer. An affected individual can never be fertile, but can lead an otherwise normal life as a woman. Oestrogen drugs can also be used to treat such individuals to create more female sex hormones in the body.

I have decided to leave this question open for those people who have this problem; you alone can decide what you want God to do for you. The decision is yours whether you want to remain a female or if you feel within you that you are a man. Once you have made that decision, then you will be able to ask God for the creative miracle you desire. Be sure of this; God wants to make you whole and to bless you, if you will dare to believe Him. God bless you. I tried several times to avoid writing on this issue but the Holy Spirit of God would not allow me such avoidance, I believe God sees your pain and wants you to come to Him so that He can make you whole. God bless you.

What the Bible offers

For those men who might have lost their penis through cancer of the penis, or who face any deformity in their reproductive organs whether what you need and desire is a creative miracle or some kind of restoration, the Word of God written below will heal, and create, and restore if applied in faith in Jesus' name.

For those men who have congenital disorders, under the guidance of the Holy Spirit, we are going into the Word of God to see what God has to tell us about congenital disorders. We are going to be dealing with the only congenital disorder on record in the Bible that our Lord Jesus Christ dealt with. I'm sure He dealt with many more, but this is the only congenital problem recorded. Using the simple truth, and the words our Lord applied to this creative miracle, you can also be made whole, as long as you behold Jesus as the great creator of the whole human race.

The Bible says:

> So I [Jeremiah] went down to the potter's house, and I saw him working at the wheel. But the pot he was shaping from the clay was marred in his hand; so the potter formed it into another pot, shaping it as it seemed best to him. Then the Word of the Lord came to me: "O house of Israel, can I not do with you as this potter does?" declares the Lord. Like clay in the hand of the potter so are you in my hand, O house of Israel. (Jeremiah 18: 3-5)

God tells us in His Word that our whole body is as open to Him as the clay is in the hand of the potter. God tells us that there is no part of our body that He cannot rebuild.

Jesus performs a creative miracle (John 9: 1-12)

> As he went along he saw a man, blind from birth. His disciples asked him, "Rabbi, who sinned, the man or his parents, that he was born blind?"

"Neither this man nor his parents sinned," said Jesus, "but this happened so that the works of God might be displayed in his life. As long as it is day, we must do the work of him who sent me. Night is coming, when no-one can work. While I am in the world, I am the light of the world."

Having said this, he spat on the ground, made some mud with the saliva, and put it on the man's eyes. "Go," he told him, "wash in the pool of Siloam." (This word means Sent). So the man went and washed and came home seeing. His neighbours and those who had formerly seen him begging asked, "Isn't this man, the, same man who used to sit and beg?" Some claimed that he was.

Others said, "No, he only looks like him."

But he himself insisted, "I am the man."

"How then were your eyes opened?" they demanded.

He replied, "The man they call Jesus made some mud and put it on my eyes. He told me to go to Siloam and wash. So I went and washed, and then I could see."

"Where is this man?" they asked him.

"I don't know," he said. (John 9: 1-12)

Be encouraged

Looking at this man, we see a man with a congenital defect; he was born blind. You may face a congenital defect or may even have lost part of your reproductive organs; be encouraged because our Lord who opened the eyes of this man, born blind, can do the same for you.

Our Lord saw him

The first thing that caught my attention in this miracle is the fact that *our Lord saw him*. Jesus himself saw this man; He saw a man who was a victim of a distressing illness, and an object of poverty and pity, a professional beggar because there were very few career opportunities open to a beggar at that time. But, on that day, Jesus saw him. He always saw quicker and further than anyone else. This beggar had stood there day by day, year after year and many people had not seen him and even those who saw had no interest in him. Even the disciples had not noticed the beggar until that day, when they saw our Lord's attention fixed on him.

But my Lord Jesus Christ always sees all. He never failed to be moved at the sight of weakness or infirmity. The Bible says that: "We do not have a high priest who does not feel our infirmities but one who was made perfect only through submission to God. He learned obedience from what He suffered. (Hebrews 5: 8) His desire always is to meet all our needs, restore all our bodies, heal and create all we need to keep us happy in this life.

So, for the man who faces congenital defects, I also want you to know that Jesus sees you, He cares about you and He loves you. His desire is to make you whole again and bring you closer to Himself.

His disciples now came out with a question: "Who sinned, this man or his parents, that he was born blind?" Jesus answered them this way. "Neither this man, nor his parents sinned, but this happened, that the works of God may be displayed in his life."

God is more than enough

Many people may come to you trying to condemn you or make you feel you are no longer a man; tormenting thoughts may even flow through your mind. Sometimes you may even feel like giving up because of the pain and hopelessness of the situation you are facing but I want to encourage you; God is more than able to heal you and restore you and give you a new beginning. He is the God of new beginnings.

I ask this question. "Does the statement made by my Lord Jesus Christ imply that the man was born blind to give God an opportunity to show what He can do with a blind man?" The question is answered by James like this: "God cannot be tempted by evil nor does He tempt anyone." (James 1: 3) "For every good and perfect gift comes from the Lord." (James 1: 17)

Congenital defects or any other problems that you may face are not God's will for your life.

Our Lord Jesus then said something else: "This happened so that the works of God might be displayed in his life." What are the works of God? Our Lord declared them thus: "The Spirit of God is on me because he has anointed me to preach good news to the poor, he has sent me to proclaim freedom for the prisoners and recovery of sight for the blind, to release the oppressed, to proclaim the year of the Lord's favour." (Luke 4: 18-19) This is the work of God; this is why Jesus left His throne in heaven and became a man; this is why He went about healing those who were oppressed; this is why He shed His blood on the Cross to redeem you and me; this is why He rose again from death to live forever more. God will not rest until all works of darkness are destroyed.

Congenital defects, or anything that brings us to the point of becoming prisoners to them, are works of darkness and Jesus has already destroyed them for us. The Bible says:

> He was despised and rejected by men, a man of sorrows and familiar with suffering. Like one from whom men hide their faces, he was despised and we esteemed him not. Surely he took up our infirmities and carried our sorrows yet we considered him stricken by God, smitten by him and afflicted. But he was pierced for our transgressions, he was crushed for our iniquities; the punishment that brought us peace was upon him and by his wounds we are healed. (Isaiah 53: 3-5)

We are already healed. No matter the congenital defect or deficiency you may face today, the Word of God says we are already healed. God laid all our sins and pains on Christ; Christ paid the price in full for all our pains and sicknesses as you can read from that passage of the Bible. Please believe this and receive this knowledge; all you need and desire has already been accomplished for you. It is up to you to receive it through faith; if you trust God's Word to be true, it will become true in your life.

The Word of God can be converted into flesh

"The word became flesh and made his dwelling among us. We have seen his glory, the glory of the Only Begotten Son, who came from the Father, full of grace and truth." (John 1: 14) The Word of God written here can be converted into flesh. What does this mean? You can, through faith, and with the use of God's Word bring about a creative miracle or restoration for whatever need you may have. "The word became flesh and made his dwelling amongst us." The Word made flesh is already dwelling amongst us - it is up to you and me what we do with the Word that is dwelling in us. We have now entered the era of creative miracles. God has shown me that anybody who dares to believe the truth from

His Word will enjoy creative miracles, no matter what that defect may be. Nothing is impossible with God.

God dwells in us

What does the word dwelling mean? A place, e.g. a house or flat in which people live. The Word of God is dwelling, i.e. living in you and me. No wonder the Bible says the Word of God is living and sharp. (Hebrews 4: 12) Only a living thing has a dwelling and God's Word is dwelling in you and me and it is up to us what we do with it. The Bible is true - God's Word is already dwelling amongst us.

Our Lord Jesus made a statement. "I must work the works of him who sent me while it is still day." This was the secret of our Lord's unwearied activity for all men. His delight was to do the will of God and to finish it. This book you are reading is part of the work that He came to do. This book is the work of Christ, not me. If you embrace the truth written in this book, you will know the truth and know for yourself that the Word of God is truth and that no Word of His is void of power.

The simple act

"He spat on the ground, made some mud with the saliva, and put it on the man's eyes." (John 9: 6) Here we see the Lord using *saliva and mud* as a means to an end. He who created the whole world only had to say a word and it was done. At other times, even without a word, miracles were performed. He said to the servants at Cana, "fill the water pots." Then we hear, "Fetch the water to the master of the feast." The next we hear is the master of the feast saying that "water" had become "choice wine." (John 2: 7) Not once did He say a word. In Genesis 1: 3, He said, "Let there be light," and there was light. But here we see Him use means.

I started questioning the Holy Spirit while walking back from my daughter's school as to why Jesus used means (saliva and mud) in this miracle. This is what He told me: "In the beginning, the Lord God formed man from the dust of the ground." (Genesis 2: 7)

What is dust?

The dictionary describes dust as fine dry particles of any solid matter, especially earth - the particles into which the body, especially human body, disintegrates or decays.

How God created man

God created man from the dust, but how many of us know nothing can be created with fine dry particles of solid matter? God needed some form of liquid to turn that dusty sand into something soft, something that could be moulded and shaped; that's where His saliva came into play. God applied His saliva to that sand and it became a soft sticky mixture of mud or clay which could be shaped or moulded.

What is mud?

The dictionary describes mud as a sticky mixture of solid and liquid, resembling soft wet earth (sand). God's saliva turned that dusty sand into mud.

What is saliva?

Saliva is described as a slightly alkaline mixture of water, protein, salt, and enzymes that are secreted into the mouth by glands that lubricate ingested food thus beginning the breakdown of starches.

God used sand and mixed it with His saliva to turn it into mud. The Holy Spirit told me that the man born blind needed a creative miracle because parts of his optic nerves were missing. On that occasion, Our Lord decided to use the same means He used to create man, to create those missing parts of the optic nerves for the blind man. When the Holy Spirit told me the man's optic nerves were missing, I just wrote it down. Later, I went to look it up since I personally did not know this or what it meant. This is what the optic nerve in man does.

The optic nerve

When a baby is conceived in its mother's womb, the genetic code governing the eye programs the baby's body to begin to grow optic nerves from both the brain as well as the eyes. Each eye will have a million nerve endings that begin growing through the flesh towards the brain. A million optic nerves will begin growing through the flesh toward the baby's eyes. Each of the million optic nerves must find and match up to its mate to enable sight to exist. The human eye has the ability to transmit to the brain over one and a half million messages at the same time. The retina at the back of the eyes contains a dense area of rods and cones that gather and interpret information presented to the eye. The retina contains over one hundred and thirty-seven million nerve connections which the brain uses to evaluate data and to attempt to interpret the scene in front of our eyes. One hundred and thirty million of these special cells are rods that enable us to have black and white vision. However, about seven million eye cells are cone-shaped cells that allow us to see colour. Each of these one hundred and thirty-seven million cells communicate directly with the brain, allowing us to interpret the visual image in front of us. Scientists have discovered that while the image we receive through our eyes is "upside down", the cellular structure in our eyes actually reverses the image to "right side up" within the eyes before sending it to the brain. The eye then transmits the corrected image at three hundred miles an hour to the brain where we "see" the image that is before us. (From the book, *The Signature of God* by J Grant.)

To me, this is the greatest miracle of all. Each day, millions of babies are born with the ability to see; their bodies have, in forty weeks or less from conception, aligned a million separate optic nerves from each eye to meet the matching optic nerve ending that is growing out from the baby's brain.

The Bible explains the intricate and skilful craftsmanship involved in making man, over 6,000 years ago, even before DNA was ever discovered.

> For you (God) did form my inward parts; you did knit me together in my mother's womb. I will praise you for I am fearfully and wonderfully made. Wonderful are your works and that my inner self knows right well. My frame was not hidden from you when I was being formed in secret and intricately and curiously wrought [as if embroidered with various colours] in the depths of the earth. Your eyes saw my unformed substance and in your book all the days of my life were written before they ever took shape, when as yet there was none of them. (Psalms 139: 13-16)

This clearly explains the intricate and complex molecules that make up the human cells. Only God could have done this. It is the work of an intelligent, loving God. He is worthy to be praised. God created man out of the dust of the earth. He mixed His saliva and dust or sand to make mud or clay and formed it and arranged it the way He wanted it to be.

The human saliva is medically proven to contain a mixture of water, protein, salt and enzymes which are secreted into the mouth by glands to lubricate ingested food, thus beginning the breakdown of starches. I believe God's saliva not only contains everything that ours contain, but it also contains life-giving power. Our Lord Jesus Christ said that the words that came out of His mouth were spirit and life. (John 6: 63)

Where do words come from? - from our mouth. Where does saliva come from? - from our mouth. The Bible says, "The tongue has the power of life and death and those who love it will eat its fruit." (Proverbs 18: 21) Where is the tongue? - in your mouth; if your body will have life today it will have to come from your tongue, in line with God's Word.

The dictionary also says that man's body disintegrates, decays into dust when he dies. God said to Adam, "...until you return to the ground, since from it you were taken - for dust you are and to dust you will return." Where does man return to when he dies? - to the ground, to dust. It is time for man to stop listening to those who cannot answer any questions about life and come back to the Bible to get the truth because God's Word is true.

Obedience

"Go wash in the pool of Siloam." (This word means Sent) (John 9: 7) The Lord after applying the mud on this man's eyes said to him: "Go wash in the pool of Siloam." So the man went and washed and came home seeing. (John 9: 9) Our Lord Jesus now tested the man's faith and gave him an opportunity to manifest obedience. The man showed faith, because he would not have acted on the Saviour's instructions. His obedience is seen as he carries out all the Lord's instruction to the very last letter. The washing was not necessary to effect the cure but doing as the Lord told him was absolutely necessary. "Whatever he saith to you, do it," (John 2: 5) is the secret of our Lord's working for us. Mary had learned that, and she was anxious for the servants to know the secret, so that the much-needed blessing would not be missed.

Obedience is the only way. When the Lord called me to do this work, I decided to obey Him, not even knowing where He would lead me. But today, as I write this book, all I can say is that I have obeyed His commands, despite many impediments - I have done all He told me to do. Nobody ever obeys Him without finding Him to be true. Many of you who need creative miracles or healing, may find that God will be giving you instructions that may be strange or unusual but, like Mary, all I can tell you today is this: "Do whatever he tells you." (John 2: 5) That is the secret of victory in everything He does for us.

Pool of Siloam (which means Sent)

The waters of Siloam in those days were sent from the temple, God's dwelling place. It is mentioned in Nehemiah 3: 15. "Shallun repaired the wall of the pool of Siloam by the King's Garden as far as the steps going down from the City of David." The Jews looked upon that pool as a kind of God's covenant with them. Today, however, we look up to Jesus Christ, the author and accomplisher of our own faith, the one who bore all our pains on the Cross, who shed His blood for us. He is sitting at the right hand of God the Father, interceding in prayers for us.

Siloam nowadays represents Christ Jesus, who was sent to us by God. To Him must all men come before they can see. He is the light of the world; He himself said, "While I am in the world, I am the light of the world. (John 9: 5) That light calls out to all men today.

For those men who face impossible congenital defects and need a creative miracle, you must come to Christ, "the sent from God". Coming to Him, you will receive total healing and restoration. Christ is the fountain opened for sin, and uncleanness, and healing, and restoration, and to Him must all men come. The blind man had eyes and could not see, nor could he when the clay was laid on him, but when he washed in the pool of Siloam - the "sent" from God - he could see.

Christ must come gushing out as a fountain before any of us can see, no matter what the infirmity may be. *Wash in - wash into*. What is washed from the man goes into the pool. How true it is that He who knew no sin became sin for us. "He bore our sin, with his wounds we are healed. The chastisement of our peace was upon him." (Isaiah 53: 5)

He was able to see - for the first time this man could see the flowers, the trees, the faces of his loved ones, his parents, the day-to-day things we take for granted. He went away and washed. He came back, able to see. Glory to God.

More than conquerors

For those men needing restoration from congenital defects that affect your reproductive system, this is what I will tell you today. This blind man came to the pool and washed. He came, he conquered by yielding to the plan set before him. Only in this same way can victory ever come to anyone, and it always comes that way. First we must go to the fountain which is Jesus Christ; there you will wash in His blood. Then we will see, and seeing, we can go out to conquer and to be more than conquerors; for the Bible says that, "In all these things we are more-- than conquerors through Him [Jesus] who loved us." (Romans 8: 37) What does "conquer" mean? It means to subdue, to master, to overcome in the sense of defeating an attack. To conquer tribulations would be to put an end to them. To conquer anguish would be to replace it with joy, to conquer famine would be to provide food. For you, today, to conquer whatever congenital defects you face would be to produce children and Paul says: "we are more than conquerors through all this, because of Him who loved us." From this scripture you can clearly see that you have more than enough to enable you through Christ, not only to conquer but to become more than a conqueror - "to him that believes, all things are possible".

This man came back seeing. You also can come back victorious. You can step out and stand out in the crowd. You can become a testimony to the glory of God. You can have that child, you can receive a creative miracle; any missing part of your body can be recreated through Christ. Why would He who did not spare His only son not give you what you need to live a happy life upon this earth? Is anything too hard for He who raises the dead? I want to encourage you to lay hold of Christ for yourself today. What He did for this man, born blind who needed a creative miracle, He can do for you. All you need to do is to ask and receive and then believe by faith that it is done. Everything else will be done by the master himself. Oh! How much he loves you, how eager he is to bless you. All you need to do is say: "Yes, Lord I believe. Forgive me all my sins, forgive me all my doubts, help thou my unbelief. Help me, Lord; I am tired. I surrender all to you." Just do this and watch what Jesus Christ will do for you. Below are some of the points of action to guide you. Most of all just come to God any way you know. The simpler, the better, if your heart is sincere. The rest is easy. God bless you.

Points Of Action

❖ Come to God through Jesus Christ

❖ Tell Him your need

- ❖ Tell Him what you want Him to do for you

- ❖ Believe by faith He has done it

- ❖ Confess it from your mouth; call it forth.

- ❖ Keep praising God until the full manifestation of all you asked is realised.

Confession

Father, I give you thanks and praise and I bless your holy name. I thank you Father that all you created is good and perfect. I thank you that every congenital problem that exists in my reproductive organs has been quickly and sharply dealt with by your Word which is creative. The Bible says You are the potter and we are the clay; through your Word I receive the creative miracle that I need in my reproductive organs in the name of Jesus. The Word of God tells me, "that Christ has already borne my pain on the cross and by His wounds I was healed." (Isaiah 53: 6). Based on your **Powerful Word** I am totally made whole.

By faith I receive the creative miracle (name relevant body part that you need) I need in the name of Jesus. The Holy Spirit of God regenerates, I thank God that His Word imparts fresh life to every organ in my body, those worn-out part of my body or those missing parts or parts that have been weakened are given a new lease of life by His powerful Word. Anything that is missing or damaged inside my body is being recreated and brought back into existence by His Holy Spirit who lives in me. The Lord daily sends me help from His sanctuary and strengthens me from out of Zion. Father I thank you for truly rebuilding the old waste places of my life. Father I thank you that you are faithful and true. I love You and I praise You in Jesus' name.

Chapter Seven

Idiopathic Infertility (infertility of unknown cause)

This is infertility from an unknown cause or unexplained. This is where all the tests and investigations have been carried out and yet no reason can be found medically as to why conception fails to occur.

The word *idiopathic* comes from the Greek word "idios", which means one's own and pathos meaning disease. Today, I would like to come into your home and just sit down over a cup of tea with you, and, with the help of the Holy Spirit, just chat with you as a couple so that I can also give you some advice that will help you.

You say to me, "Veronica, we so much desire to conceive and have children; we have spent so much money going from one clinic to another; we have done all the tests the specialists recommend, yet, when all's said and done, the doctors have told us, 'Sorry, we can't help you, since we can't find any reason why both of you cannot conceive. Sorry, we have done our best for you. We wish you well and goodbye."

You have walked out of the clinic tired, drained financially and emotionally battered, defeated, bruised; a feeling of hopelessness and defeat sweeps over you. You come home, cry in each other's arms and then you say to one another, "There is no God; if there is a God, why does He allow such pain, such suffering and misery?" You cry a bit more, and then you sit down and yet again start planning what you are going to do next.

This is where I can help.

You are a healed person

I have come here to tell you that during my research for this book, I came across so many couples who have gone this route several times and yet they are not willing to give up. They are ready to try anything. One lady actually said she would keep trying till all the money she has saved up was gone; then she would consider other alternatives. But today, I bring good news to such couples. I know the one who can help you. His name is Jesus Christ, He is the one who created you and me; He is the one who died on the Cross to set us free from sin, from infertility and every other thing that tries to bind us. The Bible says that: "He took up our infirmities and carried our sorrows; he was pierced for our transgression, he was crushed for our iniquities. The punishment that brought us peace was upon him and by His wounds, we are healed. (Isaiah 53: 4-5) You are already a blessed and healed person.

From this passage you can see that all that pain and sorrow you have gone through was not necessary. Christ has already being pierced for you; you did not need to have your body pierced again by needles etc., or undergo so much pain. He Himself had already borne your pain and by His wounds you were healed. You are a healed person. No matter what pain you are going through, please believe me when I tell you that you are a healed person. Infertility has no right to torment you, in Jesus' name. Jesus knows all things.

Jesus knows all things

The next thing I want to get clear is this statement made by the disciples of Jesus: "Now we see you know all things." (John 16: 30) Another statement that shows that Jesus knows all men is: "Jesus would not entrust himself to them, for he knew all men...for he knew what was in a man. (John 2: 24-25)

Only Jesus knows what is in a man. He knows what is wrong. He knows why you are not conceiving. He knows what to do and He is also able to correct the condition for you.

Before we continue, I will like to take us to the Bible to see a man who faced a similar situation like you, for you to see what he did. I pray that the Holy Spirit will quicken your understanding as you read this and bring you a quick victory in Jesus' name.

President decides to trust God

What would you think if the president or leader of your country came on the TV network to confess, "We in this government don't know what to do any more; we are confused and have no further sense of direction." What do you think the citizens would do? Answer that question yourself. Yet, this is what Jehoshaphat did. Three enemy armies were closing in on Judah and this mighty leader called the nation together in

Jerusalem to formulate a war plan. He needed to plan a decisive line of action. Something had to be done immediately; there was no time to be wasted. Instead, Jehoshaphat stood before his people and poured out his heart to God in confession. After praising God for His might and power, he said to God: "For we have no power to go and face this vast army that is attacking us. We do not know what to do but our eyes are upon you." (2 Chronicles 20: 12) What kind of war plan is that? - no programme, no board meeting, no war machines rolling out, nothing.

For those couples who face infertility of no known cause, I want to advise you today to stop running up and down. I want you instead to learn from what Jehoshaphat and his people did when they faced the enemy. Indeed you face a great enemy for I have already said that infertility is the enemy of God first, then of man. It is an enemy because it tries to make the command of God, which is for man to multiply, look like a lie. It is one enemy that you cannot fight on your own. You need God's help and His Word to defeat infertility.

Jehoshaphat decided to stand still, admit his confusion and helplessness in that situation, and put all the nation's eggs in one basket. They would not move anywhere but closer to their Lord; they would not look anywhere else for help but from Him.

Stop running around

I advise you to decide right now that there will be no more running up and down, no more looking to the left or to the right. You are to make a decision; today we are going to trust God; we are going to look up to Him; we are going to cast all our cares upon Him for He cares for us; we are going to put all our eggs in one basket. This time our eyes are upon you, O God. When that baby comes, Lord, it has to come from you.

What this great king did will sound stupid to most people. A lot of people today feel they must help themselves and then God will help them. The urge to make things happen has robbed many people of great victories even among Christians. Oh, we must be planning this or giving this, or doing that, or else God will not be happy with us.

Admit you are confused

This urge to make things happen contradicts the Word of God which tells us to cast our cares upon the Lord for He cares for us. He tells us to look unto Jesus, the author and perfecter of our faith. He tells us,

"Look unto me and be saved, all you ends of the earth; for I am God and there is no other." (Isaiah 45: 22) This is the biblical way to approach the problems of today. Put your hands up and say, "God, I don't know what to do but my eyes are upon you. I don't know what to do, but, Lord, you do know and I trust you to do the best for me in this situation."

Your pains and hurts

I know about all the pains and hurts you two have gone through; I know of the suffering you have gone through but I also want to tell you that God loves you. God cares about you. When you hurt, God hurts; when you cry, He cries too. For the Bible says "...in all their distress he too was distressed." (Isaiah 63: 9)

His desire is for you to reach out to Him. This is what the Lord says: "He who made the earth, the Lord who formed it and established it, the Lord is his name. Call to me and I will answer you and tell you great and unsearchable things you do not know." (Jeremiah 33: 3)

God's telephone number

When I saw this passage of scripture in the Bible, it became my favourite scripture. The God of the whole world has given me His phone number - free access to Him without any time limit. He has also promised that any hour you call, He will answer you. He has promised to show you great and unsearchable things that you do not know. Here is a definite promise to you that God will show you the cause of infertility and He will bless you; but first, like Jehoshaphat, you must call Him. You now say, "How can I call God? Where is He?" Note how Jehoshaphat called Him: "Then Jehoshaphat stood up in the assembly of Judah and Jerusalem at the temple of the Lord in front of the new courtyard." (2 Chronicles 20: 5) He was in front of the courtyard of the temple when he started speaking to God.

I want to go to the Bible to show you passages to reassure you that God is omnipresent; He is everywhere. He can hear you from anywhere you call on Him.

> Where can I go from your spirit, where can I flee from your presence? If I go to the heavens you are there, if I make my bed in the depths, you are there, if I rise on the wings of the dawn, if I settle on the far side of the sea, even there your hand will guide me, your right hand will hold me fast." (Psalms 139: 7-19)

Just call on God, It does not matter where you are, whether in the bath or in the car - anywhere; call on Him with sincerity of heart and He will answer you. As Jehoshaphat was crying out to God, He spoke back to the king and his people: "Listen King Jehoshaphat. This is what the Lord says to you: Do not be afraid or discouraged because of this vast army, for the battle is not yours, but God's." (2 Chronicles 20: 15) The king called unto his God and admitted he was helpless, then God stepped in to tell him not to worry because God Himself was the one who was going to fight the battle for him.

When you also come to God and as a couple agree that you are helpless and have decided to hand everything into God's hand, just watch and you will see what God will do for you. As God told the king: "Take up your positions, stand firm and see the deliverance the Lord will give you. Do not be afraid, do not be discouraged." (2 Chronicles 20: 17) God is saying the same thing to you - do not be afraid, my children, do not be discouraged; just take your position, stand firm and see what God will do for infertility.

What position did the king take? The Bible says: "Jehoshaphat bowed down with his face to the ground. Then some Levites from the Kohathites stood up and praised the Lord, the God of Israel, with a loud voice."

Victory through praise

Then God moved upon His enemies

> As they began to sing praises, the Lord set ambushes against the men of Ammon and Moab and Mount Seir, who were invading Judah, and they were defeated. The men of Ammon and Moab rose up against the men of Mount Seir to destroy and annihilate them. After they finished slaughtering the men of Seir, they helped to destroy one another. (2 Chronicles 20: 22-23)

Even as you start to praise God, say to Him: "Great God, creator of the heavens and the earth, I give you thanks, for your love endures forever. I thank you, for the battle belongs to you; you will destroy infertility in our home and totally annihilate it in Jesus' name, as you did to the enemies of Jehoshaphat. We worship you, O God, we praise you." As you start to praise God, watch what He will do for you.

Praise is the Christians' weapon of war. When you start to praise God, every enemy that has risen up against you flees. There is nothing that can be compared to praising God - when you praise God, every chain of bondage falls away and victory comes your way. I would advise you to emulate this. Praise is the master key into the throne-room of God. The Bible commands us to come into God's gate with thanksgiving and into His courts with praise. (Psalms 100: 4) Give thanks to His name and praise Him. If you start to praise God now for His love and mercy and start to thank Him for His faithfulness, before you know it, things will change for you like it did for Jehoshaphat when he praised God.

"Then Jehoshaphat and all the men, of Judah and Jerusalem, returned joyfully to Jerusalem, for the Lord had given them cause to rejoice over their enemies." If you do what Jehoshaphat did, the God who said "I am no respecter of person," who said "He does not change like shifting shadows," (James 1: 17), who said, "...for God does not show favouritism (Romans 2: 11), who said, "I am the Lord, I change not," will make your home a joyful place by bringing you the laughter and cry of a new baby. He is faithful.

The Bible actually says that God stoops to bless you

The Bible says ***almighty*** God stoops, to look upon those in heaven and on earth.

The seat of God almighty is so high that in order to behold the things in the heaven and on the earth, He has to humble himself, that is He has to stoop. What is to stoop? It means to bend the body forwards and downwards, sometimes simultaneously bending the knees; it can also mean to lower oneself morally. Thus the purpose of that stooping is revealed; it is so that He may raise the poor and lift the needy. Then finally the Bible moves on to say, "...he settles the barren woman..." God thus stoops again to crown womanhood with motherhood.

The God who dwells in the heights above in the heavens, stooped through His love and grace, in His only begotten son, Jesus Christ, in order that He might lift the needy. As He approached the ultimate depths in this stooping, He once again declared His intentions: "To settle the barren woman in her home as a happy mother of children." (Psalms 113: 9) Praise the Lord.

I wanted to link both these Bible accounts to encourage you to hold on to God and His Word for it is forever true. First we see God intervene in the life of a nation to fight their battle when the king and his assistants did not know what to do. If you are in the same position and you are helpless, ask God for help, He will surely step in to help you and bring you victory.

Not only will He bring you victory, He is ready to stoop down to the place where you are to bring that help. Oh, how much God loves you. Wipe your tears away and smile; the sun is shining for you today. Jesus has taken over, your victory is guaranteed. I have written down some points of action to help you as a guideline. Go to God in your own way and if you are sincere, He will surely help you. God bless you.

Points of action

- ❖ Come to God by faith.
- ❖ Tell Him about all the medical reports you have received from doctors.
- ❖ Tell Him you don't know what to do.
- ❖ Obey whatever He tells you to do.
- ❖ Believe and trust that He has done it.
- ❖ Thank Him for it.
- ❖ Confess it from your mouth.
- ❖ Keep praising God for it, no matter how the physical may look.

Confession

Father I thank you for your grace and mercy. I come to you today in the name of Jesus Christ and I bless you. I thank you that in Christ I am blessed and fruitful. Father, I thank you that infertility is far from our home; we are blessed in Christ. Our home is full of the joy of the Lord and the blessings of the Lord which include children. Today I revoke and renounce words I may have spoken into my life that may have opened a doorway for the curse of infertility to enter my life, I reject negative proclamations by parents and those who had authority over my life that may have brought a curse into my life. Every negative word that has been spoken into my life is commanded to wither and die in the name of Jesus. Every hidden disorder in my body has been exposed and quickly dealt with by the living Word of God which is powerful. I thank you, Father, in Jesus' name that I am a father of many children as you promised me in your Word.

This one thing I know for sure; if almighty God will stoop, then for sure He will bless you even more than you ever thought or imagined. God bless you.

Chapter Eight

Growths That Affect The Male Reproductive Organs

Cancer of the testes

This is a rare form of malignant tumour. It is most common among young to middle-aged men. It is most likely to happen to a man with a history of undescended testes. There are two types namely:

Seminomas

These probably develop from the cells that produce sperm.

Teratomas

This normally consists of different types of cells.

Cancer of the testes is rare and where it occurs, it usually develops from testicular tissue or from lymphatic tissue within the testes. **Symptoms:** a firm painless swelling of one testis.

Cancer of the penis

This again is a form of malignant growth or tumour that affects the penis and is more common among uncircumcised men whose personal hygiene is poor. Smoking and viral infection have been found to increase the risk.

Symptoms: A small wart-like lump or painful ulcer on the head of the penis or foreskin. It then continues to develop into a cauliflower-like mass. The growth usually spreads very slowly, but a highly malignant one can spread to the lymphatic gland in the groin in a few months causing the glands to swell, and the skin over them may ulcerate.

Any growth or sore in the penis area must be investigated immediately. Medically, if it is discovered early, it can be treated but if it is detected late, surgical removal of part or all of the penis may be necessary. There are two types of growths - malignant or benign.

What is a malignant growth?

It is a growth which tends to become progressively worse and in most cases leads to death. It spreads from its original location to establish secondary tumours in other parts of the body.

What is a benign growth?

It is a growth which does not spread throughout the body. It remains on its original site and is not life-threatening.

Spermatocele

This is a cyst (fluid-filled swelling) of the tube that transmits sperm from the testes, containing fluid and sperm. This type of cyst may start to grow or become uncomfortable. Medically, when operated on, it may result in interruption of the sperm passage into the epididymis which may render the affected testis infertile.

What is a cyst

It is an abnormal swelling filled with fluid or semi-solid material. A cyst could occur in any part of any body organ or tissue. Most times it forms as a result of abnormal activity. It becomes a growth through fluid forming in the tissue when there is no means for the fluid to escape. Cysts are harmless in themselves but in most cases, could disrupt the function of the tissue in which they grow.

I have listed above some of the problems that could happen to the male reproductive organ.

How are these growths treated medically ?

Cancer of the penis

This can be treated by radiotherapy if detected early. Otherwise surgical removal of part or all of the penis may be necessary.

Cancer of the testes

Different types of treatments are available - anti-cancer drugs or radiotherapy are also used.

Spermatocele

This will normally be removed surgically if it becomes uncomfortable but may result in interruption of passage of the sperm.

What the Bible says

Under the leadership of the Holy Spirit, we go straight into the Word of God to see what God has to say to us about these growths.

The first thing I want us to get clear is this; we normally class these growths into benign or malignant which means the one that is malignant is more difficult to treat, while benign growths are less serious; but in the eyes of God, all these growths are the same. So we will be dealing with growths from the spiritual perspective in the same way.

The principles written down here apply to both benign or malignant growths. The Word of God is not void of power and is more than able to destroy all growths once it is used in that situation in faith.

Gods fire goes into the bone

The Bible says, "...from on high he sent fire, sent it down into my bones. (Lamentations 1: 13). God's fire travels into every part of the body as you can read from this passage. It can go anywhere it is sent. It can go into the bones, into any part of the body to accomplish what it has been sent to do. (Lamentations 1: 13).

God's arm is not short

The Bible says God's "arm is not too short to rescue you, neither does He lack the strength to rescue you. By a mere rebuke, God dries up the sea, turning rivers into a desert." (Isaiah 50: 2) If God turns a whole river into dry land with one word, what hope is there for any growth to remain in your body after the Word of God has been spoken to it? I can boldly say that no growth can withstand the power of the Word of God, for the Bible says, "The grass withers and the flowers fall but the word of God stands forever." (Isaiah 40: 8)

This is how a cancerous growth or benign growth grows. Some of these growths look like plants, such as cancer of the penis which develops into a cauliflower-like mass. Some of these growths attach themselves onto a stalk and project and keep growing like stalks on a plant.

But this is what God says He will do to them. I will set them all on fire." (Isaiah 27:3-4).

God promises in His Word to set on fire any growth that tries to defy your body. While I was writing this, it suddenly came to me that even medical attempts to treat or cure these growths are made with the use of radiotherapy (which is a form of low heat energy), even though in most cases it is not successful or could lead to more damage to other cells in the body. God uses the same principle to destroy growths in the body except that God knows exactly what to do and His treatment will not destroy but preserve the human body.

God sets these growth on fire

The Bible says, "God will set these growths on fire because our God is a consuming fire." The Bible says that the mountains (growths) melt like wax before the Lord of all the earth. (Psalms 97: 5) The Bible says, "no sooner do they [growths] take root in the ground [body] than He [God] blows on them and they wither, and a whirlwind sweeps them away like chaff." (Isaiah 40: 24) You can imagine how easy it is to blow chaff away? This is how easy it is for the fire of God to consume any growth and blow it away like chaff.

For those men who face problem of cancer of the penis or testes or any other growth either malignant or benign, this is what you are to do; and if you pray these prayers then through faith those tumours will either melt like wax or wither and die in Jesus' name.

Prayer

Father, I thank you in Jesus' name. Father, I come to you in the name of my Lord Jesus Christ and based upon your Word, I rebuke all malignant or benign tumours (name growth) in the name of Jesus. I command the consuming fire of God to target these growths and melt them away like wax at the name of the Lord. I command the wind of God to sweep them away like chaff and sever their roots totally, never to grow again in my body. In Jesus' name, I cover all my body in the blood of Jesus. Now make your confession.

Father I thank you in Jesus' name. I give you praise and bless you. I thank you that any growth in my reproductive organs have been sharply and quickly eliminated from my body in the name of Jesus. The consuming fire of God has melted any growth and it will not grow again in my body in the mighty name of Jesus. Amen.

Chapter Nine

Men's Ejaculation Problems

Inhibited ejaculation

A man could find his erection is normal or prolonged but may find his ejaculation abnormally delayed or even failing to occur at all. Inhibited ejaculation could occur as a result of diabetes mellitus or as a side-effect of a long history of alcohol dependence or even treatment with certain drugs like anti-hypertensive drugs or could have an underlying psychological origin.

Retrograde ejaculation

This is where the valve at the base of a man's bladder fails to close during ejaculation. This forces the ejaculated semen back into the bladder rather than forward into the womb. This is most common among men who have had surgery in the groin area or on the prostate gland.

Where a man's sperm is the wrong shape or does not move

Some men appear to have a fault that causes their sperm to be the wrong shape or unable to move. No one knows the reason for this. It could be a result of a hormone imbalance or infection. Medically, there is very little that can be done in such cases

Where a man's body produces anti-bodies that destroy his sperm (auto-immunity)

Anti-bodies are the body's defence mechanism against disease and are produced to attack specific bacteria or virus, but at times these anti-bodies now attack a man's sperm; they make the sperm clump together and thus destroy them. Medically, treatment is difficult for men with such problems. The best that doctors can do for them is to collect the sperm, wash away the anti-bodies and then use that sperm for IVF or artificial insemination of such men's wives.

Before going any further we ask this question.

What is sperm?

Sperm is the sex cell of the male. It is also called spermatozoa. It is responsible for fertilisation of the ovum of the female. Sperms are produced within the somniferous tubules of the testes by the process called spermatogenesis. For a man to produce sperm, he must have the male sex hormone, testosterone, which is produced by the pituitary gland. The sperm is produced in the epididymis where each sperm grows a tail that will propel it through the woman's reproductive tract when the man ejaculates during sexual intercourse.

A man has twenty-three chromosomes in his sperm including the XY chromosome. This XY chromosome determines the sex of the embryo that will develop after fertilisation of the ovum.

Fertilisation

This is the coming together of a sperm from the male and an ovum (egg) from the woman. The sperm and egg unite during intercourse and an embryo starts to grow.

But as we have discussed, these men are unable to deliver their seed into their wives' wombs to start the growth of a child because of these problems. But in every situation Jesus is able.

A man said this about his ejaculation problems, "I felt like a failure."

Going through the Bible I would like to introduce you to my Lord and Saviour, Jesus Christ, and in knowing Him you will know that He alone is the sustainer of life that is ebbing away. The sign we will be looking at was given to the dying and those sorrowing because death of a loved one was close at hand; it is the same bereavement for those of you who face ejaculation problems. Jesus Christ is the one who gives life, the one who holds life, and the one who sustains life.

We go straight into the book of John to see what Jesus did for a person who faced the same problem you face. Through this problem God brought great joy and victory to the hearts of many in a home. He will do the same for you, for He is a faithful God.

Jesus, the sustainer of life (John 4: 46-54)

Once more he [Jesus] visited Cana in Galilee, where he had

turned water into wine. And there was a certain royal official whose son lay sick at Capernaum. When this man heard that Jesus had arrived in Galilee from Judah, he went to him and begged him to come and heal his son who was close to death. "Unless you people see miraculous signs and wonders," Jesus told him, "you will never believe." The royal official said, "Sir, come down before my child dies." Jesus replied, "You may go, your son will live." The man took Jesus at his word and departed. While he was still on the way, his servant met him with the news that his boy was living. When he enquired as to the time his son got better, they said to him, "The fever left him yesterday at the seventh hour." Then the father realised that this was the exact time at which Jesus had said to him, "Your son will live." So he and all his household believed. (John 4: 46-54)

First we see that out of these Galilean crowds there steps a striking figure, a man of noble birth holding an office of prominence and power. The man was probably well-known for his importance in the community, very rich and influential. We see that this man came straight to Jesus to seek help. What kind of help?

He faced the death of his only son, quite a young boy for that matter. A deadly fever held this boy in its grip. Other help must have been sought by this father for his son but without success. If money could have done it, the boy would have been healed already because it is quite clear this man was rich. But all attempts from the human side had failed to work and this father could not just stand there and see his son waste away; so the father came to our Lord and cried to him saying, "Come and heal my son, who is close to death." (John 4: 47)

For any man who faces retrograde ejaculation - where his sperm is the wrong shape or does not move - or inhibited ejaculation, there is a spirit of waste which is attacking your seed. Without help from God many men facing this problems will never be biological parents.

This father faced a hopeless situation which from the human standpoint looked totally impossible but what can man do without God? Those men who face the problems mentioned above know some of these cases are beyond any medical help. No doctor or drugs can help you. When we look at the symptoms of some of these problems we see impossibilities - man's impossibilities. No doctor or drugs can help. It is a hopeless situation. No amount of money can buy any of these things for you; most of these conditions can only be healed by God.

Next, the father heard that Jesus had arrived in Galilee from Judea - he went to Him and begged Him to come and heal his son who was close to death. If you face one of the problems described above, I want to introduce you to Jesus. The noble man heard that Jesus was in town; someone told him.

Jesus stands at the door of your heart and knocks

Today, I am also telling you that Jesus is not only in town, He is standing right at the door of your heart and is knocking, asking you to open up and invite Him to come into your life and help you. He himself said, "Because I live, you will also live; on that day you will realise that I am in the Father, and you are in me and I am in you." (John 14: 19-20) When you invite Him, as the noble man did, say to Him: "Lord, heal me."

"I have been attacked by retrograde ejaculation, inhibited ejaculation; my sperm is not moving, my sperm is the wrong shape, my body is producing anti-bodies that destroy my sperm. Lord, please help, only you can now make me a father."

You don't need to say to Him, "Lord, please come," because He is already at the door of your heart. Just ask, in simple faith, in trust and He will manifest himself to you. Say to Him, "Lord come and dwell in my heart by faith. Come and heal me, I surrender all to you."

Jesus warns against looking for signs

Jesus then said to the royal official, "Unless you people see miraculous signs and wonders, you will not believe." Why did He make that statement? Here we see a father in need and judging from our Saviour's record we see Him always ready to help the needy even when they did not ask for help. This statement was made as a stern reproof to this man and to all men, and secondly as an encouragement to these men and to all men in the world.

The desire for signs and wonders was in the spirit of the Jews in those days. The Jews required a sign. Our Lord mourns over the unspiritual state that demands marvellous manifestation before we will believe. Our generation has been caught up in this same spirit - the desire to see signs and wonders before believing.

Our Lord often gave signs to help faith, but He goes on to say "Blessed are those who have not seen and yet believe." (John 20: 29) This statement was made by our Lord as a result of an incident with one of His disciples. Thomas was told that Jesus had risen from the dead. He said to his comrades, "Unless I see the nail marks on his hands and put my finger where the nails were, and put my hands into his side, I will not believe it." A week later Jesus appeared to them again while Thomas was there. Then He said to Thomas: "Put your finger here, see my hands, reach out your hand and put it into my side; stop doubting and believe." Thomas said to Him, "My Lord and my God." Then Jesus said to him, "Because you have seen me, you have believed, blessed are those who have not seen, yet have believed." (John 20: 25-29)

Our Lord will give us signs to help our faith, but He would rather we believe Him even when there is no sign given. He would rather we take His word for what it is than build our faith on signs.

Ask and you will receive

For any man who faces the above-mentioned problems I want you to treasure in your heart this promise from God. Jesus said, "I tell you the truth; my father will give you whatever you ask in my name. Until now you have not asked for anything in my name. Ask and you will receive and your joy will be complete." (John 16: 23-24)

Let your hope be built on His words - on His promise rather than on signs and wonders. For he who believes even when he does not yet see is already blessed. A lot of times our Lord healed those who did not ask for it, but His perfect will for us is for us to ask. He loves to hear you ask Him, He loves to hear that we need Him, He loves to hear our voices, so ask Him for what you need.

The noble man's faith grew

The more the noble man was in the presence of our Lord, the more he realised that his son's life depended upon the actions of Jesus. He thought that by Jesus coming physically to his home, a cure would be effected. That was the only way for his boy to be healed - by Jesus travelling from Cana to Capernaum, to see the boy face to face.

But today I want to encourage the man who faces these problems to know that Jesus does not need to travel anymore to meet you. Christ is not limited by either time or space; He is already with you through the Holy Spirit and no boundaries of life or time can hinder His working. Even if all your sperm is dead, Jesus is the resurrection and the life. For He said, "Just as the Father raises the dead and gives them life, so the son give life to whom he is pleased to give it." (John 5: 21)

Jesus will bring life into the situation you are facing if you will dare to trust Him.

True spiritual understanding

When the noble man understood the spiritual reality of who Jesus was, he became convinced and this led him to put all his trust in the words of our Lord, even though the Lord refused to follow him home.

The test

Our Lord tested the inward sincerity of the man's faith and when he grew sincere instead of becoming angry, the desired blessing was granted abundantly, more than he had asked.

For any man facing these problems, your inward sincerity will be tested. If you are sincere, God will meet you at the point of your need, but if all you want is to play games with the Lord, you may never know who Jesus is or receive the best He has for you. You can deceive human beings but you cannot deceive Him because He looks at your heart.

Perfected faith - by His word

In that one word of rebuke the noble man was prepared for a work of power. He was not driven away, but brought nearer to the only one who could help him. Our Lord knows the human heart. He did not need anyone to tell Him what is in a man. He never tested people beyond what they were able to bear and always with the testing gave abundant encouragement. Jesus knew the noble man was in need and came to Him not merely to look for a sign; what our Lord did was to remove the father's faith from the wonder to the worker of the wonder. It does not take our Lord long to respond to the heart-breaking cry, "Sir come down before my child dies."

So no defeat or death exist in the presence of the Lord. There is hope for you through Christ Jesus. This man's faith grew as Jesus made clear to him his defects, revealing to him that true belief rests upon simple trust and obedience, rather than excitement and feelings.

Jesus said to the noble man, "No, I will not be coming to Capernaum with you but go, *your son lives*." The man did not become disappointed but his faith now rested upon the words of our Lord Jesus and he travelled home leisurely, for it was on the following day he arrived home. He did not start running home in a hurry to see if his son was still alive but he took his time. His faith was intact, he had the peace of God after Jesus spoke to him. He knew all was well. He trusted Jesus.

For the man who faces fertility problems, God's promise to you is that whatever you ask Him in the name of Jesus, He will do it for you. Will you, like the noble man, believe this promise and then relax, confident in it, knowing that His words cannot fail? When our faith is perfected, the essential request is granted.

Methods

God will always manifest Himself to us and we may not always get the answer the way we expect it, but we will always be answered. However, never believe that God will allow us to reduce Him to a recipe - that is why no one can ever predict Christ's timing and ways of answering prayers. His time is always the best and He is never late. This I have learnt myself over the few years of walking with the Lord. When you pray, leave the methods to Him; don't try to order Him around by telling Him what, when, and how to do things - it doesn't work. We can be sure He comes in time and always in His own time and way.

For the man facing fertility problems, if you have gone through fertility treatments, I know you have been told a lot about impossibilities. But today I want you to know that with God all things are possible. Don't try to figure out how and what God is going to do to help you. When you have prayed, go your way like the noble man did when Jesus told him to; do not delay for if your trust is in Him and His Word, He will be with you and guide your steps.

While the noble man was still on the way, his servant met him with the news that his boy was living. When he enquired as to the time when his son got better, they said to him, "The fever left him yesterday at the seventh hour." (John 4: 52)

For the man facing these problems, look what happens when you believe His Word; life comes back.

Life comes back into every dead situation

If you believe the Word of God, then believe that whatever you ask Him for, He has already done for you; thus, like the noble man, as you walk in faith you will find your reproductive organs perfected by a loving God and everything working perfectly for you.

Jesus at a wedding

The second Bible account I would like us to look at is found in John 2. This is an account of our Lord Jesus Christ in a wedding at Cana. Jesus at a wedding? Yes, Jesus goes to weddings, He is the God of marriage. Even today He still attends weddings where He is invited. If He is invited, He will come, He enjoys coming.

Many of us have never thought of Jesus as one who will come to a wedding to enjoy Himself. We always think of Him as one who will come to perform a priestly duty, a superior pastor, well-dressed and serious, bashing His Bible around. But that is not the Jesus I know.

Full of joy

The Jesus I know is the one full of joy who enjoys life, who delights in little children, who enjoys friendship. He enjoyed life so much that people called Him a glutton, a friend of sinners. All these were slanderous statements but the point is clear; they expected a Bible basher - what they got was a down-to-earth Saviour who loved life, who constantly cheered up people, who said to us, "Be of good cheer..." Why? - because he was happy. We have Him living in our home in the person of the Holy Spirit, as the Lord of our home, and every day we all dance as we worship and praise Him in songs; the children all have a beautiful relationship with the Lord; young as they are, they know that Jesus will always be their best friend and will always help them. The Jesus I am testifying for is real. He brings happiness wherever He is invited.

What happened at the wedding?

As this wedding progressed, the wine ran out. Jesus' mother was at the wedding also. She came to Him and said, "They have no wine." This was indeed an embarrassing moment for this couple; from all indications the couple were a bit tight on money (poor). Can you imagine the shame, especially for a young bride? I know what I would have felt if I were the one - the happiest day of a woman's life is not the day for the celebration wine for the guests to run out.

For men who face the same embarrassing situation through their infertility, I want to encourage you to "be of good cheer." No matter what the weakness is, Jesus is able to turn it into strength for you. The Bible says He works all things together for our good, for those who love Him.

Jesus' Action

In a moment Jesus had made a decision. He said to the servants who were there, "Fill the jars with water." The jars were standing nearby and the servants did as they were bid. He then said to them, "Now draw some and take it to the master of the banquet." (John 2: 6-8) They obeyed Him and did what He commanded. The master of the feast tasted the water turned into wine and not knowing where it came from, asked the bridegroom. "Why did you keep the best wine till the last?"

I would advise any man facing infertility problems to tell Jesus what problems you may be facing. In an instant, without words, He had saved this couple from shame. He can do the same for you.

The God of marriage

What Jesus did at this marriage party (feast) shows us the kind nature of God; for the Bible says that God was in Christ reconciling himself to the world. God loves weddings, God likes happiness. Here at the Cana wedding we see the eternal Christ, so human, so natural, happy in a little festive gathering of villages, empathising with the joy of young lovers in their marriage. That to me is God; that is how God feels; God is also interested in your marriage.

I want any man facing these problems today to know that God cares; He wants to come into your home, bring you joy and peace, heal you and restore dignity into your life, bless you with children and even more. The Cana couple ended up rich that day. Jesus left them with 180 gallons of choice wine, which they could sell and so start their married life together with money made from the sales. That is how thoughtful our Lord is. When He comes into your life, He brings super abundant blessings. Read more about this revelation in my book, *Woman, You Are Not Infertile,* in the section on congenital disorders.

Invite Him anyway

If you face infertility because of the problems I have outlined above, I would like to encourage you to invite God into your marriage. Marriage is not child's play. Without God as the third party in a marriage, it could become stale - unprofitable, unkind, and unloving. Having been married for some years now, I can testify that without Him I do not know what I would have done. His constant presence has sustained both my husband and I, and our children during trying times. No amount of love is safe without God in it. After the partying is over, after the honeymoon, when the blinds are drawn, only God can make a difference in a marriage because He is the God of marriage. He is the one who instituted marriage and knows best how it should work.

Today, invite Jesus into your home, into your situation and let Him bring you joy and peace. Remember He loves and cares for you. These are some of His promises to you.

> I will uphold all those who fall and lift up all who are bowed down. (Psalms 145: 14)
>
> I will open my hands and will fulfil the desire of all living things. (Psalms 145: 16)
>
> I will watch over the way of those who fear me. (Psalms 145: 20)

That is the God you are calling. He is faithful.

I want to link both Bible accounts together to encourage you to trust in the Lord and to know that He cares for you. In the first account, we see a noble man who faced the death of his only son. No human being alive could help him, no money could buy back the life of that boy; but Jesus came into that situation and brought joy and peace back into it. We see Him at the wedding turning water to wine to save a young couple from shame and embarrassment; in both cases we see the Lord intervening in family life, to make sure that joy, peace and honour were retained.

In your case, you mean much to God too. His desire is to come into your home, heal you, and leave you with joy and blessing as He did for this Cana couple, if only you will invite Him into the situation you are facing and trust Him to bring victory to you.

Points of action

❖ Come to God by faith

❖ Tell Him all areas of medical report you received from doctors.

❖ Ask Him to heal you.

❖ Obey and do whatever He tells you to do.

- ❖ Believe and trust He has done it.

- ❖ Thank Him for it.

- ❖ Confess it from your mouth.

- ❖ Keep praising God for it, no matter how things may actually look.

This one thing I know, "I know that the Lord saves His anointed. He answers him from His holy heaven with the saving power of His right hand." (Psalms 20: 6). God bless you.

Confession

Father, in the name of Jesus'I give you praise and I bless you. I thank you that all ejaculation problems are far from me. I know that beacause I dwell in the secret place of the Almighty I will continue to rest in His shadow and with confidence I can say of the Lord, He is my Refuge, my Fortress, my God in whom I trust." The Father has totally healed my body from all ejaculation problem and disease and has bestowed abundant life on me. I thank you Lord because you promised that whatever I ask the Father in your name you will do for me. I ask you Father for beautiful and healthy children today and I thank you in advance because I know that it is done. God grants me abundant prosperity so that when I lie down none shall fill me with dread or make me afraid; God has removed savage beast from coming within my dwelling place. The sword of evil will not pass through my home. I pursue my enemy ejaculation problem and it has fallan by the sword before me. God looks on me with favour and makes me fruitful and increases my numbers. He keeps his covenant with me. While my wife is still recovering from last year's childbirth, it is time to make room for even more babies. God loves me. He walks with me. He has destroyed the yoke and bars of ejaculation problems and has blessed me with healthy children with my head held high. (Leviticus 26:3-13). The Father is rebuilding the old waste-places of my life, I'm like a green pine tree; my fruitfulness comes from the Father. (Hosea 14:8). All that the canker worm have eaten the Father is now restoring to me. He is like the dew to me. He makes me blossom like a lily, like a cedar of Lebanon, He makes my loin blossom and produce strong and healthy babies. Thank You Father in jesus' name. Amen.

TYPES OF INFLATABLE PENILE IMPLANTS

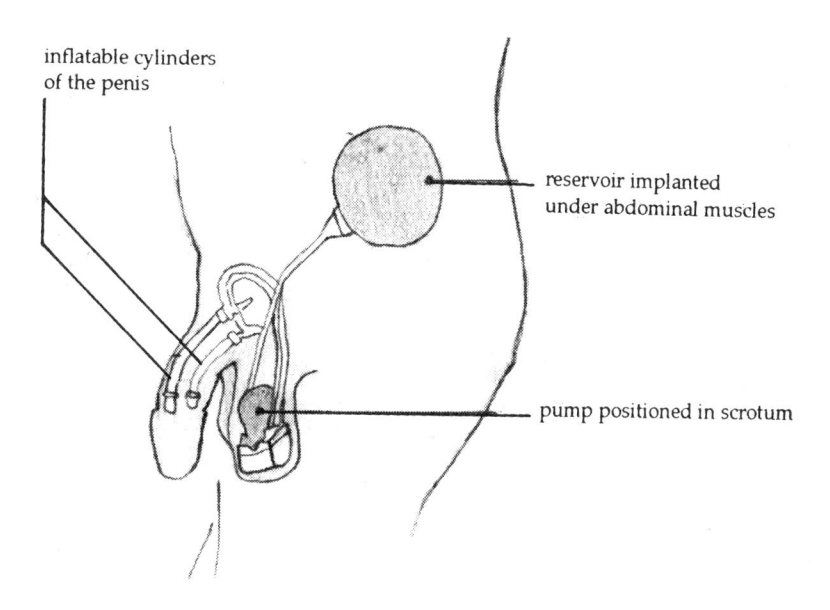

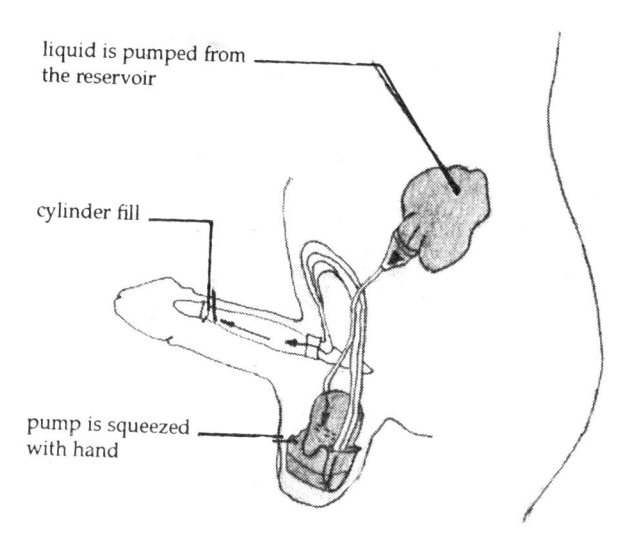

inflatable cylinders of the penis

reservoir implanted under abdominal muscles

pump positioned in scrotum

liquid is pumped from the reservoir

cylinder fill

pump is squeezed with hand

HOW VESECTOMY IS PERFORMED

This operation is normally performed to block the passage of the sperm from the testes.

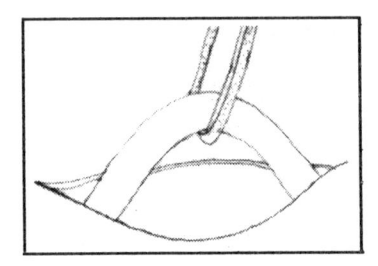

1. An incision will be made on both sides near the root of a man's penis: Then the sperm tube, the vas deferens is cut free of the spermatic cord. No blood vessel is cut.

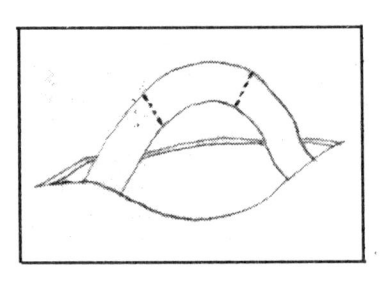

2. A loop of the vas deferns is freed and then brought out of the incision. From this stage there are several possibilities; usually a length of the vas deferns is cut off.

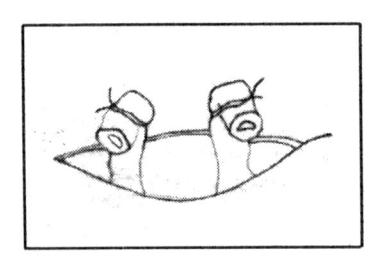

3. To prevent the cut vas deferens from rejoining, it will often be bent back and tightly closed with ligatures. Once this is done the tubes are pushed back into the spermatic cord.

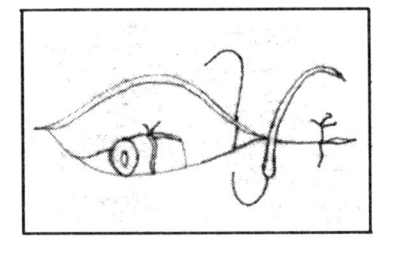

4. The incision made is closed up with three or four sutures. The man will experience a mild pain for a few days.

X and Y Chromosones

Female

female cells contain two X chromosomes

all eggs contain X chromosomes

if an X-containing sperm fertilises the egg, a female embryo starts to grow

Male

male cells contain one X and one Y chromosome

sperm cells either contain one X or one Y chromosome

if a y-containing sperm fertilises the egg, a male embryo starts to grow

ANATOMY OF THE SCROTUM

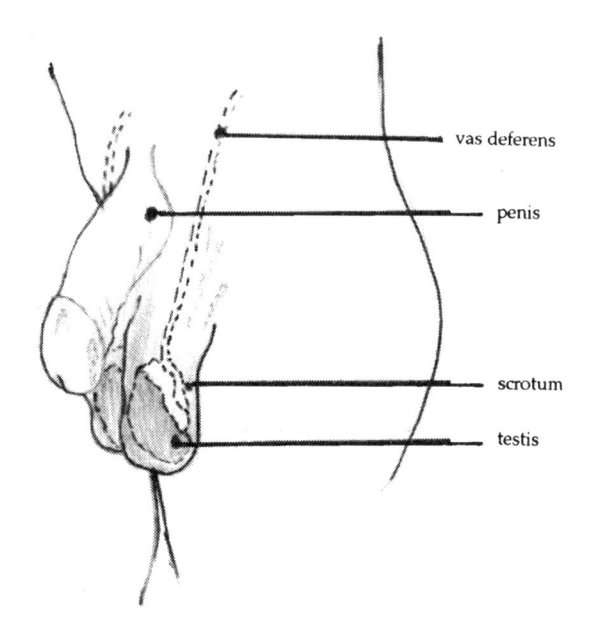

- vas deferens
- penis
- scrotum
- testis

A SPERM

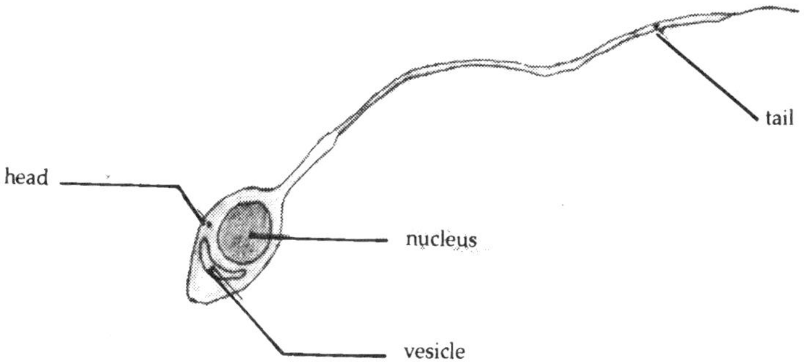

head
tail
nucleus
vesicle

During love making a man will normanally ejaculate between 500-800 million sperms,most of which are capable of fertilising an oveum. But, as they travel upwards (propelled by their whip-like tails), more than half are killed by acidic vaginal secretion; many more die during the journey up through the cervix and womb and into the fallopian tube.The journey can take from one to five hours, and in the end, only a few thousand survive.

THE JOURNEY OF THE SPERM

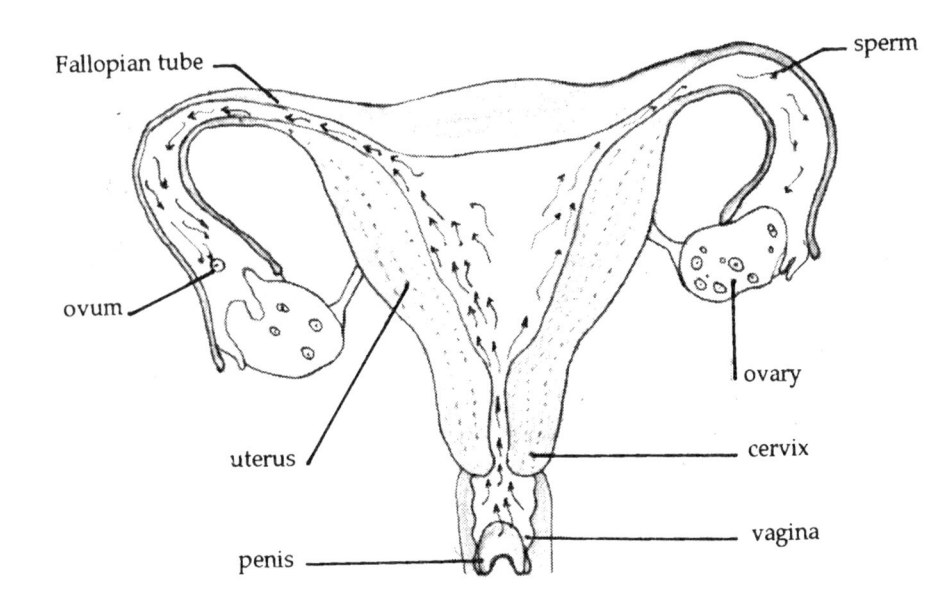

- Fallopian tube
- sperm
- ovum
- ovary
- uterus
- cervix
- vagina
- penis

A Sperm can live in a Fallopian tube for up to 48 hours, during which time it is capable of fertilizing an egg.

MALE REPRODUCTIVE ORGAN

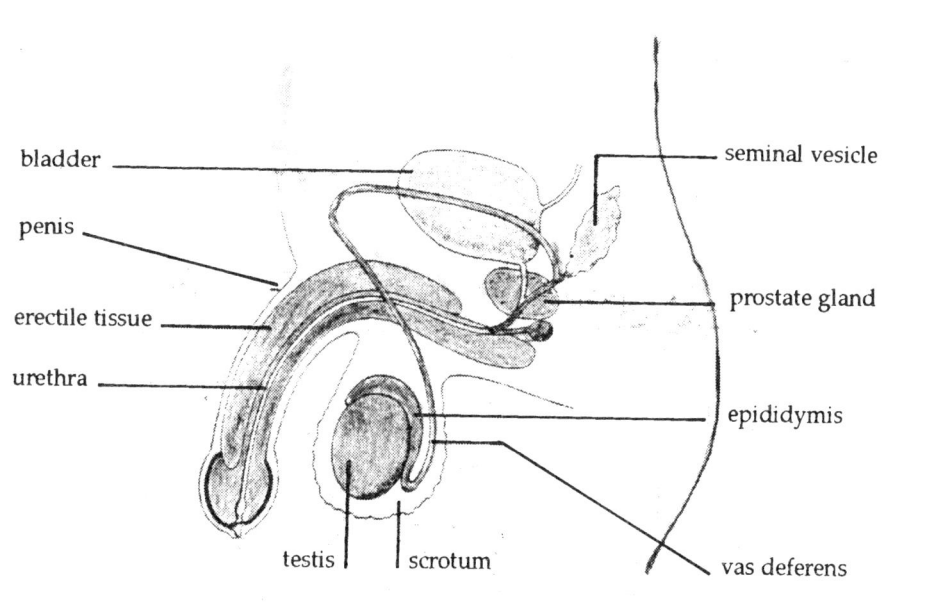

- bladder
- penis
- erectile tissue
- urethra
- testis
- scrotum
- seminal vesicle
- prostate gland
- epididymis
- vas deferens

Chapter Ten

What The Word Of God Can Do In Our Life And Body

For the Word of God, "... is living and active, sharper than any double-edged sword. It judges the thoughts and attitude of the heart, it penetrates even to the diving soul and spirit, joints and marrow. Nothing in all creation is hidden from God's sight. Everything is uncovered and laid bare before the eyes of him to whom we must give account." (Hebrews 4: 12-13).

For the Word that God speaks is alive and full of power (making it active, operative, energising and effective). It is sharper than any two-edged sword, penetrating to the dividing line of the breath of life (soul) and (Immortal) spirit and of joints and marrow (of the deepest parts of our nature), exposing and sifting and analysing and judging the very thoughts and purpose of our hearts. And not a creature exist that is concealed from His sight, but all things are open and exposed, naked and defenceless to the eyes of Him to whom we must give account (Hebrews 4: 12-13).

The Word Of God Is Powerful

God's Word is powerful and covers a lot of problems and other things we meet or face from day to day. It is still:

Alive:

Having life still in existence, in force or in operation, active. The Word of God has life in it. Our Lord Jesus Christ said, "the words that I speak to you they are spirit and life." He came to the grave of Lazarus, a man who was dead four days and He called out in a loud voice "Lazarus, come out," and the dead man came out. His hands and feet were still wrapped with strips of linen and a cloth was round his face. But our Lord's words were put to action and it worked. (John 11: 43-44)

Active:

Characterised by practical action rather than by contemplation or speculation. The Word of God takes an interest and makes quick physical movement. It is lively, marked by vigorous activity, it is practical and is capable of taking an action on its own initative when activated. The Word of God does not waste time contemplating or speculating on what to do. Rather It takes a quick intrest in the situation and quickly apply practical solutions to it, bringing in a quick, active and positive change into that situation.

Sharp:

Adapted to cutting or piecing, e.g. having a thin, keen edge or fine point. Keen in intellect, perception, attention. Capable of action or reacting strongly. Cutting in language or implication. Affecting the senses or sense organs intensely. Clear in outline or detail. The Word of God is sharp and can be used in a situation where a tumour or growth needs to be sharply cut away from an organ of the body. Because of its sharp nature, it is capable of performing an operation and cutting through any form of growth or disease without any damage to the organ involved or risk to the life of the person it is operating on.

Quick:

Fast in understanding, thinking or learning, mentally agile, reacting with speed and keen. Fast in developing or in occurrence, for example a succession of events done or taking place with rapidity. Marked by speed, readiness or promptness of physical movement. Inclined to hastiness, e.g. in action or response to find fault. Capable of being easily and speedily prepared.

This I have experienced time and time again. While writing this chapter, I went shopping one evening and while coming back I was singing and praising God, and along comes this old man, shuffling along with his dog. He stopped and said to me: "Why are you so happy?" I replied that my happiness was about Jesus Christ who fills my heart with joy. He asked me to tell him more about Jesus Christ, because He was a good man but did not know who Jesus was. I stood there and explained to him who Christ is. He decided He wanted the Lord Jesus Christ in his life. I prayed with him there and he received salvation. He told me he had no kneecap and had endured six operations on his back and was due for the seventh one. I laid my hands on him and prayed for him and I asked God to create new kneecaps and heal his back. In less than the few minutes it took me to pray for him, he could bend down which was something he could not do before. I praise God for that.

The Bible says the Word of God is quick, fast in understanding, thinking, reacting with speed and keen in sensitivity. Marked by speed, and rapid physical movement, while doctors are busy taking x-rays or all sorts of tests, the Word of God has quickly and speedily finished off what needs to be done, because it takes a quick interest in any situation and quickly and promptly brings a solution to it.

Exposed:

To deprive of shelter or protection, lay open to attack or influence. To subject to an action or influence, to subject to action of radiant energy. To lay open to view, to display, e.g. to exhibit for public veneration. To bring shamefully to light.

The Word of God exposes every hidden thing. How many times have you seen a sick person tell you they are sick and yet after medical investigation no one can detect what is wrong with them? Not so with the Word of God. The Word of God deprives disease of shelter in our bodies. He lays every hidden sickness open for attack and subject to the power that is in His Word. He stripes open to view every hidden disease, bringing it shamefully to light.

Judges: A judge forms a judgement or opinion about any given situation. The Word of God is a judge. God left His Word on earth to be judge for us in all life situations. Who is a Judge? A judge is somebody who judges, e.g. a public official authorised to decide questions brought before a court. Somebody who gives an authoritative opinion. The Word of God is able to form an opinion, to make a decision as soon as it is applied to a situation. It is able to give an authoritative opinion on every issue or situation in life. Be it physical or spiritual, because it is a Judge. This is a good scripture for those with infertility of unknown cause, the Word of God judges and quickly gives a decision on the issue. And the decision is always based on the truth of Gods Word.

Living:

The Word of God has life in it. It is alive.

Operative:

Producing an appropriate effect. The Word of God exacts power or influences situations or factors operating against us. It influences sickness, disease, or anything standing in the way of our success. It produces a desired effect.

The Word of God performs surgery. Yes, the Word of God is capable of performing major or minor operations, without the person being cut or suffering any pain. The surgery done is to bring about or cause any organ or part of our bodies to function, or be put in normal operation the way God ordained it to function in Jesus' name.

If we put our faith into action and believe God, He will surely make what we are beliving Him for come true.

Energising:

To give energy to, to make energetic or vigorous, to apply energy so as to facilitate normal operation. The Word of God energises. The Word of God is able to give energy, make vigorous any situation or any part of the body that could be dead. It is able, when applied in faith, to bring back life and facilitate normal operation of any part of the body that may be impotent - you can, by applying the Word of God, receive life back in any affected part of the body, or any life situation that needs a resurrection.

Analyse:

To subject to analysis, to determine the constitution or structure of a thing. The Word of God is able to analyse any problem and form an immediate opinion about it.

In the next chapter we will be using the analyses from the word of God to bring healing to those who face infertility of unknown cause.

Chapter Eleven

How to avoid unnecessary tests and treatment when having difficulty in conceiving

If you as a couple have being trying to conceive for more than a year without any result, if sexual intercourse has been taking place normally and no pregnancy has resulted, or if you suspect either of you have a problem not yet identified by the doctors and you desire to avoid all the hassles of infertility treatment, this is what you can do. I'm not advising you not to go to your doctor, please, but any man who has gone through all fertility tests will tell you that it is not a pleasant experience. However, what you do is your personal choice and decision.

Here is my suggestion to you based on the Word of God. You have to speak to your body. Remember the chapter on the power of your own words. The Bible says, "...the lips of the wise protect them," (Proverbs 14: 3) which means that if you choose to be wise now, you will protect yourself from suffering and pain, and save the thousands of pounds that infertility treatment will cost you. The Word of God says that the tongue that brings healing is a tree of life (Proverbs 15: 4), which means your own words can bring healing into your body when you line them up with God's Word. Let's look at the medical investigation you will undergo when you go to the fertility clinic for testing.

Men

The first test for investigating male infertility is semen analysis. If such a test reveals that a low sperm count is present, more tests may be needed to investigate what the underlying cause might be.

Semen analysis

Semen produced by masturbation is examined as soon as possible for the number, sharpness and degree of mobility of the sperm.

A post-coital semen test may also be performed.

Abnormal sperm

There may be present in the semen large numbers of abnormally shaped sperm, such as the two-headed ones which may reduce a man's fertility. We now go straight to the Word of God and we are going to be selecting from the analysis of Hebrews 4: 12 as to what the Word of God does for our bodies.

Men's confession

Father, I thank you in Jesus' name. I give you praise and honour, Father; I put my trust in your Word and I apply your Word to all parts of my reproductive organs, commanding them to work properly in Jesus' name.

The Word of God to become operative and effective

Penis:

I speak to my penis and I say to it, "Failure to achieve and maintain an erection is bound in the name of Jesus; abnormal ejaculation or any hidden disorder that exists is bound in Jesus' name. I command my penis to operate, to keep working and to function normally and remain effective by producing a baby in Jesus' name.

The Word of God to energise

Testes:

I speak to my testes in Jesus' name; I say to them if you are producing few sperm or none, or if my sperm are abnormally shaped, too short-lived or have impaired mobility, I command them in the name of Jesus to hear the Word of God. God's Word energises, it gives energy to facilitate normal operations. I decree that my testes are working normally, producing healthy sperm in the name of Jesus.

The Word of God is to become powerful

the Vas Deferens:

I speak to all the organs within my penis, especially my Vas Deferens, saying that if any structural abnormality exists that could impede the passage of my sperm, I apply the powerful Word of God and, in the name of Jesus, command the Word of God to perform surgery to put everything in working order, In Jesus' name. Amen.

As you apply these principles from the Word of God to your reproductive organs, they will perform their specific duties and become healed where necessary. Before you know it, your beautiful wife will definitely be pregnant; in Jesus' name.

Good news! While the book was being edited I gave this prayer to a couple who have been trying to conceive for some years. Within eight weeks they were pregnant. It works. Just do it.
God bless you!

My prayer for you

Father, in the name of Jesus Christ, I pray for this couple under the authority you have given me; I pray that as they confess your Word into their bodies that your Word will bring light and dispel darkness. I stand in agreement with them that you will grant them the desires of their heart. In Jesus' name. Amen.

Chapter Twelve

The Power Of God's Word -And The Power Of Your Own Words

The Word of God cannot fail

One of the attributes of God's Word is it's infallibility. The Bible says Heaven and earth will pass away but not a *tittle* of God's Word will fail. God said the "words that come out of my mouth will not return void, but accomplish the purpose for which they are sent," (Isaiah 55: 11) - which means God's words will never return to him empty. No! They will always accomplish their purpose and that is why I advise you today, that if you agree that any word you read here is the Word of God, and you apply it in your situation, it will surely accomplish that which it is meant to accomplish.

The Word of God is alive

Jesus said that the words which I speak to you are both spirit and life. That means every Word of God is already power-packed, carrying with it the power to manifest itself. God does not need your help or mine to let His words be fulfilled. All He requires from us is to trust (have faith) that what He has said He is able to bring to pass. Obedience is also important on your part. God may ask you to do things which may look or seem stupid to the ordinary man but obedience will lead you to inherit God's promises. (Isaiah 55: 8-9) says that "God's way is not man's way and God's thoughts are not man's thoughts - His ways are higher than our ways and His thoughts higher than our thoughts." You can boldly say to yourself that because God's Word carries miracle working power, the fulfilment of your need is not in you but it is in God's promise to you.

The Word of God creates

The Word of God does not only heal but it can create whatever parts of the body you may be missing or needing. Read in John 1: 14 : "The word became flesh." This is so important for those needing creative miracles. The very word you have received concerning your need can be converted so that it becomes flesh - this work will be done in your spirit and the manifestation will appear in the physical as a creative miracle, in the area of your need. For example, in Genesis 1: 3, God wanted light and said, "Let there be light," and there was light. The Word God spoke quickly turned into flesh and manifested itself into light. Let's take, for example, the possibility that you need a new penis or vas deferens. You can call it into flesh by the Word of God spoken out of your own mouth and it will become flesh - tangible in your life.

> For God said from now on I tell you of new things, of hidden things unknown to you. They are created now and not long ago; you have not heard of them before today. (Isaiah 48: 6-7)

From this you can clearly see that God is still creating new things because he is able to create.

The Word of God sanctifies you

Our Lord Jesus Christ prayed this prayer for us -Sanctify them by the truth; your word is truth. (John 17: 17) What does the word "sanctify" mean? it means to be set apart for a special purpose or sacred (Holy) purpose.

Every man is set apart by God for a special purpose as a precious instrument through which God can bring a child into the world.

God watches over his Word to see that it is performed: (Jeremiah 1:12)

What is to watch? it means to keep guard, to keep awake during the night especially to keep vigil, to be closely observant of an event or action, to watch while alert or to guard or to protect closely; that's what God does over His words. He hovers over them like a mother hen hovers over her chicks. He who watches over *Israel* (you and me) will neither slumber or sleep. (Psalm 121: 4) Can you imagine that your God does not sleep but is watching over all the words he has spoken to you until they are performed? His words can be totally trusted and depended on.

The Word of God sustains everything on earth

"The Son is the radiance of God's glory, and the exact representation of His being, sustaining all things by His powerful Word." (Hebrews 1: 3) We can see clearly that the Word of God is what is ruling the world today. God created this world with His Word and is still sustaining and running everything with it. You and I, everybody, is subject to God's Word and everything, including infertility, and all human problems must bow to the Word of God.

The Word of God is the remedy for impossible situations

The Word of God can be used in all situations. Because of its infallibility it is the only remedy for impossible situations in the world today. "For what is impossible with man is possible with God." (Luke 1: 37)

THE POWER OF YOUR OWN WORDS

Having discussed the power of God's words, we will also go into the Word of God, to see what God has said about our words. I also want you to know that the greatest battle you will ever face is not infertility. The greatest battle you have to fight is getting your words in line with God's Word, to bring about your miracle.

Everyone, created by God, has the ability to express themselves, their plans, thoughts, perceptions, heart's desires, and visions, through words. God has given us the ability to express our innermost desires through words.

Why?

This is what the Holy Spirit taught me.

> The Lord God formed the man from the dust of the ground, and breathed into his nostrils the breath of life, and the man became a living being. (Genesis 2: 7)

What is dust? The dictionary says that 'dust is fine, dry particles of any solid matter, especially earth.' They are the particles which the body disintegrates or decays into when it is buried.

God created man from the dust as the Bible says, but how many of us know that nothing can be created with fine dry particles of solid matter? God needed some form of liquid to turn that dusty sand into something soft, that could be moulded and shaped. That's where His saliva came into play. God applied His saliva to that sand, and it became a soft, sticky mixture of mud or clay, which could be shaped or moulded.

The human saliva is medically proven to contain a mixture of water, protein, salt and enzyme, that is secreted into the mouth by glands that lubricate ingested food, and it often begins the break-down of starches. I believe God's saliva not only contains what ours contains, but it also contains life-giving power. Our Lord Jesus Christ said, "The words that I speak to you, they are spirit and life." (John 6: 63)

Have you ever wondered why Jesus spat on the ground, made some mud with the saliva and put it on the eyes of the man born blind? (John 9: 6)

God's saliva gave life to the human flesh

The saliva came from God's mouth. It gave life to the flesh, because it contained life in it. Then when God breathed into the man's nostrils with His mouth again, the life in the saliva ignited together with the life in His breath, and man became a living being.

God programmed your body to respond to His Word

Now, this is the interesting part. God programmed every part of man to respond to His Word. Because His saliva is in every part of our bodies, therefore, every part of our bodies must respond to the Word of God. Our bodies actually hear, understand and obey God's Word, because the Creator programmed each part with His saliva in order to give life to it.

When the body hears the Word of God, it responds and obeys it, because God has programmed it that way. The Bible says (in Proverbs 18: 21), "The power of life and death is in the tongue." Have you ever really thought about these words? God has put the power that holds your life in your mouth. If you are to succeed or fail in life, it is going to be up to you. You hold the power in your tongue to build your life, either for death or for life. It is up to you.

You can programme yourself by the Word of God. When you feel as though you are falling sick, instead of accepting it, you can say to yourself, "What does the Bible say about this?" It says, "By His stripes I am healed." (Isaiah 53: 5) If it looks like that baby is not going to come you can look at what the Word of God says: "In Christ I will bear much fruit." Therefore you don't say what the circumstance is saying. You say what God says. Your body hears and sooner or later it will line up with the Word of the Manufacturer Who programmed it to work and run perfectly on His Word. What will happen to a car if you fill the tank up with water? That is exactly what many of us have done to our bodies. God has left us the manual (Holy Bible), telling us the Manufacturer's instructions for use and the remedies in case of emergency, but all we have done is ignore it, and run up and down looking for help where we can't find it.

The Bible says:

> The mouth of a righteous man is a well of life. (Proverbs 10: 11)

> The mouth of the just bringeth forth wisdom, but the forward tongue shall be cut out. The lips of the righteous know what is acceptable. (Proverbs 10: 31, 32)

A righteous man is supposed to know what is acceptable. In our speech, what God said is what is acceptable. When you begin to quote what God said, it will just be as though God said it Himself. It will work for you like it worked for Him. If you programme your spirit with God's Word, and do not doubt in your heart, but believe that those things which you are saying will come to pass, they will come to pass.

Do you believe that the baby will be born? Do you believe that missing chromosomes can be re-created? Do you believe that sexual organs can be re-created? If you believe, start to say it now. Our Lord Jesus Christ made this statement about our speech.

> I tell you the truth, If anyone says to this mountain, Go throw yourself into the sea, and does not doubt what he says, it will be done for him. (Mark 11: 22)

This is a fact. It is the law of the Spirit. It can never fail, because it is the Word of God. This statement speaks for itself. If you face anything which is lacking, which has caused infertility in your life, by saying what the Word of God says, you can turn it around. Jesus Himself said that you can have what you ask for, whether good or bad.

Whatever miracle you desire today, you must confess it from your mouth. It may not manifest itself today or tomorrow or next week, or next month, but if what you are saying lines up with the Word of God, it must surely come to pass. At times it may look like there is no change.

It may look like nothing is happening. It may look like God is not hearing you, but I can say today, if you stand on God's Word, it will surely come to pass.

When you confess it, some may laugh at you. Others will think you are stupid, but please don't listen to anyone. Keep your focus on God and His Word.

Jesus Christ is the High Priest of our confession (Hebrews 3: 1)

Christianity itself, is a confession. When you confess, you confess with your lips. What do we confess? We confess the "finished work of Christ for us." We confess that He is seated at the right hand of the Father, having redeemed us from the penalty of sin. We confess that He has, "Blessed us with every spiritual blessing in the Heavenly Realms in Christ. (Ephesians 1: 3) We confess that we are healed already. These are the things you are to confess. God has promised us this:

> Peace, peace to him who is far off and to him who is near! says the Lord, I create the fruit of his lips and I will heal him (make his lips blossom anew with speech in thankful praise. (Isaiah 57: 19)

God has promised that He will create the fruit of your lips. So what do you want created? Make sure that is what you are confessing or saying from your mouth. And God will bring it to pass.

In concluding this chapter, this is my advice to you. Please don't go around telling people all your troubles to get their sympathy. It will not help you. Cast all your cares on the Lord, because He cares for you.

Telling people all your problems, only makes you lose faith with God, and puts you in doubt. But saying what God's Word says, in spite of every circumstance, brings faith into your heart. The living Word of God on your lip makes you a victor, makes infertility and disease your servant - it brings God on the scene - brings victory and joy and success.

Example of a person who did not watch his words

> Zachariah and his wife had prayed for years to have a child. Finally God sent an Angel to tell him his wife was going to conceive and have a son. When the Angel told him his wife was going to have a child, Zachariah asked the Angel, "How

> can I be sure of this? I am an old man and my wife is well on in years..."
>
> The Angel answered, "I am Gabriel, I stand in the presence of God, and I have been sent to speak to you and to tell you this good news. And now you will be silent and not able to speak until the day this happens, because you did not believe my words, which will come true at their proper time."
>
> Meanwhile, the people were waiting for Zachariah and wondering why he stayed so long in the temple. When he came out, he could not speak to them. They realised he had seen a vision in the temple, for he kept making signs to them, but remained unable to speak. (Luke 1: 18-22)

Here we see God take an extreme action to shut a man up, for the Bible records that throughout Elizabeth's pregnancy, Zachariah was unable to speak.

> On the eighth day, after the child was born, they came to circumcise the child, and they were going to name him after his father, Zachariah, but his mother spoke up.
>
> Then they made signs to Zachariah to find out what he would like to name the child. He asked for a writing tablet, and to everyone's astonishment he wrote, "His name is John. Immediately his mouth was opened and his tongue was loosed." (Luke 1: 59-64)

Here God bound Zachariah's tongue so that his prayers might be fulfilled and that the favour of the Lord might be upon Elizabeth, as God had spoken. As soon as this came to pass, God loosed his tongue. I am sure God took this extreme measure because Zachariah could have killed this miracle with his mouth, because the Bible says the power of life and death are in our tongue. And the child born was so important in the plan of God for the world.

Many of you carry seeds of great destiny, so watch your words in order that God's favour may rest on you and your family. Remember, the power of life and death are in your tongue.

Chapter Twelve

Let's Talk About faith

What is faith? It is an allegiance to duty or to a person, loyalty, for example in good or bad faith; fidelity to one's promise, a belief and trust in and loyalty to God or the doctrines of a religion, complete confidence and a strong belief with strong conviction, especially of religious belief. Today in the world, we have a lot of religions and people put their faiths in these religions but today the faith I am writing about is the faith based on the gospel of Jesus Christ.

Faith to me simply means trust in God. What is to trust? It means to put confidence, to depend, and to hope and to do without fear or misgiving, to rely totally on God. When you trust God, you are able to rely completely on him; you depend on him and you permit him to direct your course in life without fear or misgiving.

The Bible says that, "without faith, it is impossible to please God because anyone who comes to him must believe that he exists and that he rewards those who earnestly seek him." (Hebrews 11: 6)

Before you come to God, first you must accept that he exists, then secondly you must also believe that he rewards those who earnestly seek him. The Bible says that the same Lord is Lord over the Jews and Gentiles and rewards those who come to him.

In discussing faith in God, we are going to be talking about Abraham, the father of faith. Abraham had a promise from God when he was an old man and this promise reads "I will bless Sarah and will surely give you a son by her. I will bless her so that she will be a mother of nations. Kings of people will come from her." (Genesis 17: 15-16)

"Even though Abraham did not know how such a promise could come to pass, his faith grew strong and he did not worry about the fact that he was a hundred years old and that Sarah, his wife was ninety years and was too old to have a child." They never doubted but they believed God and their faith grew stronger and they praised God even before the promise was fulfilled, being sure that God, who gave the promise, was able to bring it to pass.

Finally, the Bible records that, "now the Lord was gracious to Sarah as he had promised and the Lord did for her what he had promised. Sarah became pregnant and bore a son to Abraham in his old age at the time God had promised him and Abraham gave the name Isaac to the son that Sarah bore him." (Genesis 21: 1-3)

Abraham and Sarah had survived the physical limitations placed on them by the laws of nature which said they were too old to be parents; now they had a son because they stood by their faith in the promises of God.

After the boy was born, God then came in to test Abraham. This is where Abraham became the father of faith and sealed his eternal blessing and destiny to inherit God's promise which said that it is through him that all nations of the earth will be blessed.

The test itself

God said to Abraham, "Take your son, your only son, Isaac whom you love and go to the region of Moriah, sacrifice him there as a burnt offering on one of the mountains of which I will tell you." Early the next morning Abraham got up and saddled his donkey. He took with him his two servants and his son Isaac.

When he had cut enough wood for the burnt offering he set out for the place God had told him about. On the third day Abraham looked up and saw the place in the distance. He said to his servants, "Stay here with the donkey while I and the boy go over there. We will worship and then we will come back to you." (Genesis 22: 5)

Abraham continued alone with the boy to the designated place with the wood for the burnt offering and gave it to his son Isaac who carried it while Abraham carried the knife and fire. Isaac spoke up and said to his father, "Where is the lamb for the burnt offering?" Abraham answered, "God himself will provide." Abraham got to the mountain, prepared the altar for the burnt offering, lay the boy on it and then he reached for the knife to slay his son. But the angel of the Lord called out to him from Heaven, "Abraham! Abraham!" "Here I am," he replied. "Do not lay your hands on the boy," he said, "Do not do anything to him.

"Now I know that you fear God, because you have not withheld from me your son, your only son." Abraham looked up and there in a thicket he saw a ram caught by its horns. He went over and took the ram and sacrificed it as a burnt offering to the Lord.

"Take thy only son and sacrifice him as a burnt offering." This is the greatest test of faith any human being can face. Abraham had waited 100 years to have this boy, all his love and hope and dreams were built around this boy, his heir, the one who was to live after him, maintaining God's promise which God had promised Abraham. This was Isaac, Abraham's laughter, the one who brought back joy into his life and now the person who had given him this boy was asking for him to be offered as a burnt sacrifice.

What did Abraham do? - he obeyed God

Abraham rose up early in the morning and went as the Lord commanded him. He obeyed God. He carried out in detail every instruction given to him by God. For the Bible records that when, "They came to the place which God had told him of; Abraham built an altar there, and laid the wood in order and bound Isaac his son, and he laid him upon the altar upon the wood. And Abraham stretched forth his hand and took the knife to slay his son. All this clearly shows Abraham reaching the ultimate in obedience.

Why this level of obedience?

Abraham said to the servants: "Stay here with the donkey while I and the boy go over there. We will worship and then we will come back to you."

Abraham was leaving his two servants behind, he was going away to build his altar, going away to slay him, going away to give up his only begotten son. He and Isaac were going away to worship. YES, but he said, "We will come again."

His faith rested in God's abilities

In Hebrews 11:17 we find the answer. "By faith, Abraham, when God tested him, offered Isaac as a sacrifice. He who had received the promise was about to sacrifice his one and only son, even though God had said to him, 'It is through Isaac that your offspring will be reckoned.' Abraham reasoned that God could raise the dead, and figuratively speaking he did receive Isaac from the death." (Hebrews 11: 17-19)

Abraham "reasoned that God was able to raise Isaac up, even from the dead." Abraham was walking in obedience to God, to give up his son in whom all his hopes were centred, the son of his love, he was going through with it at all costs, but believing that God was able to raise him up, even from dead". He "reasoned", he was arguing, arguing within himself, and on the basis of his argument, was coming back to a definite conclusion.

Looking back to God's faithfulness

Abraham was looking back to where God had brought him from. Knowing how Isaac came to him at the age of 100 years old, he was saying to himself, "I will obey God at all costs. I know God cannot fail to keep his promise, and if I, in obedience slay my son, then God will raise him up from the dead rather than fail, either in His promise or His purpose." Abraham's reasoning was based on the knowledge he had gained of God by the previous revelation he had received from God. All his past experience had prepared him for the line of argument which is the argument of faith.

Note his words to the servant "me and the boy will worship, and we will come back to you." Note his answer to his boy's question "where is the lamb for the burnt offering?" "God himself will provide the lamb for the burnt offering, my son." Abraham had full assurance he would be coming back with Isaac but how it would be done was what he did not know. He also knew by faith that even if he slew Isaac, God would be able to raise him from death; for God had said to him, "it is through Isaac that your seed will be reckoned." Abraham saw with the eye of faith; the eye of faith always sees beyond the physical eye.

His hope was built on God's Word and promise; his faith was built on the action which resulted from reason, through the recognition of God. His faith was built on God's promise, not on Isaac. Abraham believed God. He believed God's Word to him. The Bible records that this was put into his Heavenly account for righteousness. What will you want to be deposited in your Heavenly account? Faith or fear? Look at Abraham's faith and decide for yourself; the decision is yours.

My personal journey of faith

What a journey it has been for me! I met the Lord Jesus Christ on the 27th of August 1992 and I also met the Holy Spirit the same day. That became the happiest day of my life. I had found what I was looking for. The empty space in my heart was filled. I had found the owner of the empty space, his name is **JESUS CHRIST!** My life was never to be the same again. During this period I was facing a great trial in my life and someone invited me to church and I said yes. That was the best decision I ever made.

After meeting the Lord in that service, that first day, I had the assurance that everything will work out well in my life. I told the Lord all I was going through and he gave me the assurance that everything would be all right. I thought it would be the next day, but it wasn't until nine and half months later that the promise came to pass. It's wonderful! During this period of waiting for God's promise in my life, my faith grew.

How did my faith grow?

I spent a lot of time in prayer, going to church, investing money in good Christian books, tapes, audios and Christian magazines. I also developed my relationship with the Holy Spirit. Within three weeks of knowing the Lord, I was praying for the sick on the road and in the bus and the Lord was confirming His Word by healing them on the spot. This encouraged me a lot and helped my faith in God to grow.

A little girl's eyes restored

This is probably one of my happiest testimonies. I sat in church one Sunday morning with a pretty girl and her mum right in front of me. This baby was less than a year old; she was very beautiful. I did not know that she was blind in one eye as a result of cancer. During that service the pastor at my first church came in and asked that we pray for the little girl. It was then I realised that the little girl was sick. We prayed for her recovery in December 1992. She was due for her check-up in January 1993 when, if the cancer was still there, the eye would have to be removed. She went back to hospital in January 1993 and the cancer had spread. Immediately she was operated on and the eye removed.

Meanwhile I could not get that girl's picture out of my mind. I started praying for her telling the Lord that baby was too beautiful to be blind, telling God it was not His will for her to remain blind. I cried before the Lord for some weeks I did not see that family again after that first meeting.

After some time, I forgot all about the family and did not pray any more. Then one day in March 1993, I was in the bath when the Lord said to me, "Remember the little girl with the cancer in her eyes. You were praying for her. I heard all your prayers and I am going to heal her today." I said. "Lord, I don't know their names or their address or where they live." I called my former church to find out their details. Nobody knew anything about them any more, because they were in the hospital.

God moves supernaturally

When I finished all my phone calls and no one seemed to know their name or whereabouts, the Lord dropped the name of the hospital and their name in my spirit, and told me to go. I waited till the evening to get someone to go with me to the hospital because all these experiences were a bit too much for me.

When we got to the hospital, we asked for the children's ward and were directed to it. We walked into the ward and the first person we saw was a lady, and we walked up to her. I quietly mentioned the name the Lord had given me to this lady and asked for the family.

It turned out the lady was her doctor. She was the one treating that baby. Immediately I spoke the name, she said, "Oh! That blind girl that had her eye removed." From that encounter, the Lord led me to that little girl. When I told the mother how I got to her, she could not stop crying. She said to me, "I have been crying out to Jesus. I knew he would not forget me." We all cried and then we prayed.

I laid hands on that baby and we left. There was no immediate change, but within two weeks that baby was totally healed and her eye that was removed was totally restored by the Lord. The last time I saw her, she was perfect, and growing happily. She was able to see with both eyes .

This probably helped me on my journey of faith. I knew that God can do mighty things in our lives and through us if we dare to trust him. Going to that hospital that day was a trying of my faith. I did not know this family's name or even if they were in that hospital but I obeyed the voice of my Lord and Saviour Jesus Christ. That obedience saved the life of a little girl.

I have so many testimonies I could share on this journey of faith but I will stop here for now. My personal life has been tested and tried time and time again but I have put my trust in God and His Word and His promises to me. I refuse to worry because I know God has been faithful and will continue to be faithful to the end.

What I Have Found Faith To Be

After a few years of walking with the Lord all I can tell you is that I have found faith to be" trust" in God and His Word.

If God says He will do it then I believe it and apply this knowledge to my life. If God says he has done it, then I accept it and apply this to my life. I have tried and proved the Word of God and I can tell you it is "*true*"; that which I am writing to you today is all true. If you want to see God's power don't try to reason things out, like wondering how it can be done, leave that to God. Figuring it out only brings confusion. Leave it to God as He said: "Cast your cares upon me for I care for you." God will always come true for you. Every thing else may fail but God's Word and His promises can never fail.

I have found faith to be the currency of Heaven; there is nothing you cannot buy with the faith that is focused on Jesus Christ and God Almighty.

What if my faith is weak?

Weak faith considers the problem instead of the promise of God's Word. Don't spend more time with the problem than with the promise. For every problem, there is a promise.

Many of you reading this book may never have heard of Jesus Christ before today. Reading about faith you may be saying, "Oh, I have no faith!" You may not even be sure of what I am talking about.

I want to encourage you to be of good cheer. In whatever place you find your yourself today, God is able to come down there and meet you and then bring you up one step at a time, for there is room for growth in the body of Christ.

The example I am going to use to demonstrate weak faith is also about Abraham and his wife Sarah. The Bible so exalts Abraham's faith but I want to bring something out of this - the Word of God is balanced. It is true! Before Abraham became the father of faith he had no faith at all.

When God came to Abraham to reconfirm his covenant with Abraham, this is the conversation that took place between them.

> God also said to Abraham, "As for Sarai your wife, you are no longer to call her Sarai; her name will be Sarah. I will bless her and will surely give you a son by her..." Abraham fell face down; he laughed and said to himself, "Will a son be born to a man one hundred years old?"

Then Abraham trailed off in another direction:

> "If only Ishmael might live under your blessing!" (Genesis 17: 15-18)

Ishmael was the son he had by a slave woman. Abraham did not believe God here.

Sarah

She laughed the first time God's promise came to her, that she would be a mother of many nations. Sarah laughed and said to herself: "After I am worn out and my master is old will I have this pleasure?" Neither of them believed God's promise the first time.

Once again Abraham almost blew all God's promises to him in Genesis 20.

> For a while he stayed in Gerar, and there Abraham said of his wife Sarah, "She is my sister." Then Abimelech, King of Gerar sent for Sarah and took her. But God came to Abimelech in a dream one night and said to him, "You are as good as dead because of the woman you have taken; she is a married woman." Genesis 20: 2-3

God stopped Abimelech from going near Sarah and Abimelech did not sleep with her. God then told the king to return Sarah to Abraham and asked Abraham to pray for him; so that the king would live. (Genesis 20: 7)

> Early the next morning the king summoned all his officials, and when he told them all that had happened, they were very much afraid. Then Abimelech called Abraham in and said, "What have you done to us? How have I wronged you that you brought such great guilt upon me and my kingdom? You have done things to me that should not be done." And Abimelech asked Abraham, "What was your reason for doing this?" Abraham replied, "I said to myself, 'there is surely no fear of God in this place, and they will kill me because of my wife.'" (Genesis 20: 8-11)

This reply was given by Abraham to King Abimelech to explain why Abraham deceived him that his wife Sarah was his sister. Here we read of Abraham's:

Departure from faith

Abraham the father of faith departs from the path of faith to walk a path of deception and lies. In his departure from walking by faith we see him making arrangements for his own safety through deceitful practices, in that he told the half-truth that his wife was his sister, she being his half sister, the daughter of his father, Tera, by another wife. The sad thing about this is that he had done this before during his visit to Egypt.

Abraham thought that among a people who lacked the fear of God, he must act for himself, and without God. God knew from this experience that Abraham pretended to have fear when it suited him; and therefore that it was not only unnecessary, but also wholly wrong, for him to act as he had done.

By such action he had placed the whole purpose of God in jeopardy, and, but for the intervention of God, it would have been made impossible of realisation through Abraham. What foolishness we get ourselves into whenever we try to limit God in our thinking, and thus have to fall back upon our own policies! To act thus is always to turn aside from the higher ways of his purpose and to imperil the possibility of working together with him. God now intervenes in this issue by making Abimelech return Sarah, Abraham's wife, to him unharmed. Thus God did not allow Abimelech to sleep with Sarah, Abraham's wife.

The point I am making here is that no matter how weak your faith may be today, if you come to God and trust in Him and start to read the Bible, your weak faith will start to grow and as it grows you will start to exercise it and it will also increase as you exercise it.

Abraham went through all these trials initially but his faith grew to the point where he was able to become the father of faith, where he was able to sacrifice his son without withholding him from God. In Abraham's journey with God he started with very weak faith, but he continued to grow in faith, till he got to the point where he was ready to sacrifice his only son, ready to obey God at all cost.

How do you grow in faith?

The Bible says that " faith comes by hearing and hearing by the Word of God. That means faith must have been somewhere before. Since it comes, faith is in the Word of God. You can receive faith by hearing the gospel preached, by listening to the Word of God, by reading good Christian books, watching videos and listening to audio tapes.

All these activities help faith to come into your heart. And as it comes it grows. The Bible says that Abraham, even though he was past the age and Sarah herself was barren, was enabled by faith to become a father because "he considered him faithful who had made the promise." (Hebrews 11: 11)

Today if your heart's desire is genuine, and you desire to know God and trust him, he will give you ample evidence for faith and he will help you come to the light. You must be honest to God and to yourself for the Bible says that the Holy Spirit helps our weakness; when we do not know what or how to pray he helps us. The psalmist wrote: "Teach me to do your will, for you are my God. May your good spirit lead me on a level ground." (Psalms 143: 10)

The holy spirit will lead you and teach you as long as you remain open and honest to God. Through your relationship with the Holy Spirit your faith in God will grow.

When I ask God for something in faith how many times must I ask?

A lot of people usually advocate asking God till you receive what you desire. Personally I have walked with the Lord almost four and half years now. I have never asked him for anything that is specific twice. What I do is ask once and then start to praise him for it. I believe God hears the first prayers and answers the very first time. The physical manifestation may take a while but while waiting I mount up on the wings of praise, remind God of His Word from time to time and thank him for His promise. I tell Him that I believe He has done it and that when the time is right He will bring it into the physical.

I have followed this pattern and it has worked for me. I pray that you will cultivate your relationship with the Holy Spirit so that he will teach you what will work best in your life. If it a specific prayer I believe asking once is enough. There are, though, areas which I believe are right for continuing prayer - where prayers are ones such as for those in authority, the success of our pastors, leaders, our spiritual growth, daily protection. But outside these areas I personally believe you should ask once, then remind God again from time to time in an attitude of praise rather than asking again and again, e.g. "Father, thank you for all

I asked, [mention what you asked] I believe you have done it, it is just a matter of time before I see it in the physical. I bless you, because I know at the right time you will bring it into the physical. I know you have done it in the spirit and I bless you for it in Jesus' name."

Keep reminding God of the promise as recorded in His Word and keep praising Him. In due season He will bring it to pass.

How to focus your faith; be specific in what you ask

Your faith must be clearly focused on a goal. For the Bible says faith gives substance to the things we hope for. (Hebrews 11: 1) The prayer of faith leads us to see visions of what we desire. The Bible says Abraham did not believe by looking at his own body which was dead at one hundred years old. Instead Abraham and Sarah saw their children by faith and that's how they were able to receive the promise. You must see it before you receive it.

Begin now to see a little baby in your arms by faith. The God who helped Abraham and Sarah to see the impossible will help you also see your own baby in Jesus' name, for the Lord never changes.

Watch your words. Keep your confession right and get rid of obstacles that may negate your prayers. Let your words be in line with your prayers. Keep praising God and thanking him. Read your Bible, listen to the Word of God and let your faith grow. When the time is right God will bring all you have asked Him to pass. Hold on to God and be strong, for our God is powerful and merciful. God bless you.

CHAPTER FOURTEEN

Giving

Today, in writing about giving, I would like to introduce you to the greatest giver of all. He is God Almighty. The Bible says that, "God so loved the world that He gave His only begotten Son." (John 3: 16)

Have you ever imagined what it cost God to give His only Son to redeem the world from death? I guess this is one thing we all can never understand. At times when I talk to people about the death of Christ, they just ask questions like, "Was it necessary for Him to die for us? Why did God not just kill Satan instead?" These questions are good questions, but the truth of all this is this; if it was not necessary God would never have crucified His Son.

Today in the body of Christ, giving has become a controversial subject. Many people don't like talking about it; they have their own ideas about giving which has nothing to do with Christ. The people that complain are the same as those who will go to a fertility clinic and pay thousands of pounds for a treatment that may never succeed. If you did not pay that money the fertility clinic will have to shut down their business for lack of money; this is the same with the gospel of Jesus Christ. The Word of God is free, but those who preach the gospel need finance as well to pay church bills ,electricity bills, etc. What will you say if you got to church on a winter's morning and there is no heating because the bills have not been paid? If you are sitting in a cold church you will not be able to hear the Word of God properly. So for the effective preaching of God's Word we must learn to give. Personally, this book will not be complete without my advising and telling you the truth about giving.

If you read through all the Bible accounts I used in my book on infertility, you will notice that all the people who God blessed were those who loved to give or even vowed to give. I am not saying God will not bless you because you did not give. But there are certain levels of blessings attached to giving.

Manoah and his wife

The first couple we are going to be talking about is Manoah and his wife. In Judges 13 is the Bible account of Manoah and his wife who were sterile: barren. The angel of the Lord came to this couple and told them they were going to conceive and have a son. After the angel gave them instruction on what to do, then

> Manoah said to the Angel of the Lord, "We would like you to stay until we prepare a young goat for you." The Angel of the Lord replied, "Even though you detain me, I will not eat any of your food. But if you prepare a burnt offering, offer it to the Lord. (Judges 13: 15-16)

This couple not only loved God, they knew how to worship God. They would not let the angel of God go without giving God what they could afford. Notice that God did not ask for this offering, but this couple decided to offer it.

When they offered this sacrifice, as he and his wife watched, the flame blazed up from the sacrifice towards Heaven, "the angel of the Lord ascended in the flame." (Judges 13: 20)

God accepted this offering of thanks. It was pleasing to Him and that sealed their blessing.

My personal experience of giving

I also want to share my testimony on giving to encourage you to give to build the body of Christ. For the Gospel of Jesus Christ to spread all over the world, it is going to need those who are committed to sacrificial giving.

The first day I gave my heart to the Lord, the Lord lead me to buy three books that totally changed my life, and laid a foundation for my Christian walk. One of these books was *Dream Seed* by Mike Murdock. In this book I learnt some of the most powerful principles of giving in my life. The very next Sunday, when I was going to church, I went to the bank and took out some money I had saved. I put that money in an envelope and dropped it in the offering basket, to be used for the work of God.

After that Service, we went to a brother's house with his family and my friends. While there we were praying and that was when God came to me and made me this promise. He said to me, *"Veronica, because of that offering you gave today, the blessing I have for you will flow like the widow's oil. You will not have room to store it.* (2 Kings 4)

I started weeping with joy, because I was happy that my offering was acceptable to God. Up to this time of my writing, I have not yet stepped into the widow's oil blessing physically, but I believe that spiritually I have stepped in there, because I feel it stirring up in my spirit. Four years down the road, I can boldly write and say, I have sought the kingdom of God with all my heart. Everything I could give to build the body of Christ, I have given. God has also been faithful to me. Not once has He withheld any good thing from me. His blessings have remained upon my life. I can boldly say that I have been faithful to God; be it in tithe or offering, God has always been first. I also believe God will bring His promise to pass, because He is a faithful God.

Many of you reading this book may be needing great things that you want God to do for you. I can boldly tell you, when you give, you honour God. You show Him that you care. Each time you open your hand and give to the Glory of God something leaves God's hand to bless you.

Anyone who loves gives. God loved us, He gave His only Son. God keeps giving. No one can out-give God. Please get this clear in your spirit; everything you have comes from God, but God still desires that we take a part of what He has given us to worship Him. Whatever you give is used to build up others less privileged than you. It is used to bless the poor or preach the Gospel.

What you give is not directly given to God in the sense that He has a need. *No!* God has no need. For the whole world, and everything in it belongs to Him, including you and me.

But He has laid down the principle of sowing and reaping and giving and receiving as tools He uses physically to bring blessing into our life. Have you ever wondered how a farmer sows a handful of seeds and in a few months reaps a harvest which is greater than the handful of corn he sowed? So it is with sowing into the work of God. Your handful sown will return in a great abundance of harvest, for the Bible says, "whatever a man sows he will reap." (Galatians 5: 7)

The lady with the oil

We now go to meet the lady whose sacrificial giving preserved the body of Christ.

> It was two days to the Passover and the Jews' Feast of Unleavened Bread. Jesus was in Bethany, sitting at the table in the home of a man known as Simon, the leper. A woman came with an alabaster jar of very expensive ointment (perfume) made of pure nard. She broke the jar and poured the perfume on Jesus' head.
>
> Some of those present were saying indignantly to one another, "Why this waste of perfume [or ointment]?" It could have been sold for more than a year's wages, and the money given to the poor." And they rebuked her harshly. "Leave her alone!" Jesus said. "Why are you bothering her? She has done a beautiful thing to me. The poor you will always have with you and you can help them any time you want. But you will not always have me. She did what she could. She poured perfume [ointment] on my body beforehand to prepare for my burial. I tell you the truth, wherever this Gospel is preached throughout the world, what she has done will also be told, in memory of her."
>
> Then Judas, Iscariot, one of the Twelve, went to the chief priests to betray Jesus to them. (Mark 14: 1-10)

Before I go any further, I would like to take the time to write in honour of a great lady, who loved her Lord and gave the best she could to preserve the body of Christ. In this very first work I have done, I have chosen to obey the command of my Lord, Saviour and Master, Jesus Christ. This is His command to all ministers of the Gospel.

> "I tell you the truth, wherever the Gospel is preached throughout the world, what she has done will also be told in memory of her."

What did she do?

Our Lord said it Himself, "She hath done what she could; she is come aforehand (beforehand) to anoint my body to the burying." (Mark 14: 8)

She came into that house with a jar of ointment. What is *ointment*? - the dictionary says it is a soothing or healing salve for application to the skin.

What is perfume?

It is a sweet or pleasant smelling fragrance; a pleasant smelling liquid.

What does the word anoint mean?

It means to smear or rub with oil or a similar substance; to apply as a sacred rite; to consecrate, to prepare, to declare or make sacred.

She came into the house with a jar of pure nard used by the Jews for embalming dead bodies.

What is to embalm?

To treat a dead body so as to give protection against decay.

Preserving the flesh of Jesus

She started anointing Jesus on his head. She poured that perfume on His head, but from the words of our Lord, "She came to prepare my body for burying", we know she made sure that oil went all around His body, from head to toe. She anointed Him. She consecrated Him. She declared that she has prepared His body for burial.

Why?

Has it ever struck you that nobody pours embalming oil on a live person. This oil is used for preserving the body of a dead person, yet she poured it on Christ. Why?

If you notice, after she anointed Jesus, Judas, one of His disciples, went from that room to the Chief Priest to betray Jesus to them. (Mark 14 : 10) From that anointing, Jesus went to His trial and then to the Cross. He never had an opportunity to take a bath, after She anointed Him.

When He left that room, He was smelling like death already. He was alive, but was already embalmed, prepared for death.

Why did she do this?

When Jesus came into the world, God had to conceive His flesh in the body of a woman. Then the Spirit of God had to dwell in the flesh of Jesus. Now Jesus was about to die; God had to preserve the flesh of Jesus Christ from decaying in the grave. I heard that in the Middle East where Jesus lived, the dead has to be buried immediately; if not, their bodies started to rot and smell immediately. Please remember Jesus was a man in human flesh like you and me. Even though He raised Lazarus from the dead, He was the resurrection and the life while He was there, but now He had to die to be able to resurrect all who will ever die again in this world. He was dying for the sins of the whole world. His flesh had to go underground for three days. God knew what He was doing. The Spirit went into the kingdom of darkness to destroy the works of darkness, but the flesh was in the grave.

His flesh was needed again

As we read in the Gospels when Jesus rose from the dead, His Spirit came back into the flesh, because the flesh had been preserved from decay, and many witnesses saw Him again, before He finally went up to Heaven to be with the Father.

The woman's boldness

For what this Jewish woman did that day, she needed Holy Ghost's boldness to be able to do it. Here all these men were seated in a room, but she boldly walked up to our Lord Jesus Christ and did what God had commanded her to do. She prayed, she was sensitive to being led by the Holy Spirit into knowing exactly what to do. She was a woman on a mission. When you meet a woman on a mission, you will always detect boldness in her.

Open rebuke

The disciples rebuked this woman. They called what she did stupid and senseless. They did not know any better. Yet what she did that day was in the plan of God.

Many of you will be mocked when you give, but please don't listen to those people who want to stop you from giving. You never know what your giving will accomplish.

God needs your body too

Today God is saying, "I need your body to be able to preserve the body of Christ." You may say, why?

Legal authority given to man (meaning male and female)

When God created the earth, God gave it to man, as we read (in Genesis 1: 26), God made man and gave him authority to "rule over the fishes of the sea and the birds of the air, over all the livestock, over all the earth."

So when man sinned and broke faith with God, God had to devise a plan to be able to bring Jesus down to earth as a legal person to be able to bring man back to Him. A spirit needs a body to operate through.

For anything God will accomplish on earth, He will need a man to co-operate with Him and the Holy Spirit to be able to accomplish that thing. Today, God is looking for a man or woman who will say yes to His plans and purpose.

A year's wages

The men who rebuked the woman said she wasted a year's wages worth of oil. This woman did not bother with them. She knew what she was doing. They did not.

Today, God is calling you and me to help preserve the body of Christ that the Gospel be preached around the world. Money is needed. First, you must plant the seed with the little you have, then God will use the little seed to give you an abundant harvest for you to put into His work.

Have you ever wondered how a handful of corn is planted and a few months later, abundant crops are harvested. That is how it is with God. What little you plant, He will give it back to you in abundance. God needs you to obey and give to build the body of Christ, like the lady with the oil. Do not be afraid to give. Nobody can out-give God.

Eternal blessing

This woman's giving established an eternal blessing. You and me, and many more coming into the kingdom of God today, must appreciate what she did on that day, to preserve the body of Christ.

Remember that you never know what your giving will accomplish in the kingdom of God. But obey God and give anyway.

Everyone has something to give

Many of you may say, "I have no money to give to God's work. I have nothing to give." But today I want to tell you, if you really want to give, you have something to give. If not money, you can give your time, to the glory of God, by serving in the church, and helping the needy. When I asked God for a son in 1994, I gave him back to God even before I conceived. I told the Lord to give me a son, who will be a man of prayer in His kingdom when he grows up. Today, to the glory of God, my son is almost five years old now, but nobody can stop him praying. He is always praying. So you see, if you are faithful, God will be faithful. Even when you are unfaithful, God remains faithful.

The lady with the oil gave her best, a year's wage of perfume, to prepare the body of Christ. I personally cannot even put a figure to the amount I have sown into God's work in the past few years, but I can boldly say, I have given all that I could without holding back.

What will you choose to do today?

Remember the great lady who anointed Jesus' body to preserve it from decay - Jesus memorialised her giving, commanding every preacher of the Gospel to do this: "Wherever the Gospel is preached throughout the world, what she has done will also be told in memory of her." (Mark 14: 9) We are to tell the whole world what she did. She preserved His body.

You may never know what your giving will accomplish, but give anyway. Forget the critics - those who will not give and love to discourage others from giving. Obey God and see what God will do for you.

Where do I give?

Where you sow your money matters a lot. Let us take, for example, a vineyard owner who must plant his vine on a suitable and well drained hill to be able to have a grape harvest. Grapes will not grow on just any ground, so also it is with your giving. I would advise you to give to your church, if you go to church. If not, I would suggest that you ask the Lord to direct you to a ministry or a good cause of his choice, and then send whatever you desire to give to them. God will bless you as you do that. Even if you don't give, God will still bless you when you believe His Word.

Points of action

- ❖ Be specific and ask God what you desire.
- ❖ Believe by faith that you have received it.
- ❖ Determine in your heart what you want to give to God.
- ❖ Make sure it moves you.
- ❖ Be faithful to fulfil it.
- ❖ Look for a good soil to sow your seed.
- ❖ Keep praising God; at the right time your seed will bear fruit. God bless you.

Chapter Fifteen

Major Questions On Infertility Answered From The Bible

Question: What are the spiritual causes of infertility?

I noticed whilst researching for this book that, medically, little is known about infertility. This got me questioning the Holy Spirit about it. He taught me quite a few things which I have added in this book. Why did I desire to do this? As you read through the pages of this book you will notice it is full of miracles and restoration, but at the same time I must present to you a balanced Gospel. The Gospel of Jesus Christ is balanced; His promises to His Children are many and all are victorious but on the journey to victory are also warnings of great afflictions. "Many are the afflictions of the righteous but the Lord delivers him out of them all." (Psalms 34: 19)

Jesus told us about all the good things that he had in store for us, but he also painted a total picture to prepare us for every situation in life. There are many reasons scattered throughout the pages of the Bibles as to why infertility happens to many people even among born-again Christians. This is because someone could be born again and still operate under a curse. "Infertility is a curse of the law." Until that believer learns to take authority over it. Deuteronomy 28: 18 reads like this: "The fruit of your womb will be cursed," as the price of sin and disobedience but Galatians 3: 13-14 says that "Christ has redeemed us from the curse of the law by becoming a curse for us, so that the blessings given to Abraham might come to the Gentiles through Christ Jesus and by faith."

If you, as a child of God, desire to be free from infertility you must take a stand. If there are areas you need to deal with in your life deal with them and then take a stand. Having children is God's greatest desire for man. Procreation is of God, it is God's main reason for creating us.

Imagine if all people on earth, especially Christians, were barren, soon we would have ended up without witness. God blesses us with our own children who will spread the Gospel and bring God's love to the world from that family after their ancestors have died. That is why the Bible says that "a good man will always leave an inheritance to His children's children." (Proverbs 13: 22) Why?

Because that is God's greatest desire. God alone dreamt up child birth and then created us with that desire in us. The Bible says that God himself desires Godly offspring. (Malachi 2: 15)

Before infertility is experienced in the physical it has already started in the spiritual realm which you and I cannot see into. All of life's battles are won or lost there. Then we experience victory or loss here on earth. Nothing written here is to judge anyone, but it is written so that if anyone finds themselves caught up in any of these situations, there could be a turning around and forsaking of those things so that God's blessings can rest upon you. There is no point praying for a child and then not dealing with the issues that could have led to the problem in the first place, that of lack of conception. May the Holy Spirit help you to grasp the truth and run with it in Jesus' name. Amen.

God shuts the womb

At times God himself shuts the womb, waiting for a specific time to bring a special child into the world. The Bible says in Acts 17: 26 that God himself determines the times set for every human being to be born and the exact place where they should live. Even down to parents, location of place of birth, God alone determines it all. The Bible says that there is "a time to be born." (Ecclesiastes 3: 2) Only God determines that time.

Medically, after nine months of pregnancy comes birth. What triggers birth? Nobody knows. Doctors know that the baby, not the mother, makes the decision, but there are no clues as to how that decision is made, but the Bible has answered this question for us.

"He [God] determined the times set for them [all men coming into the world] and the exact places where they should live. (Acts 17: 26) The Bible asks this question of us - Is he (God) not your Father, your creator, who made you and formed you? (Deuteronomy 32: 6) Yes, He is.

Through the guidance of the Holy Spirit we now go to the Bible to see examples of when God shut the womb.

Hannah -(I Samuel)

In I Samuel we read of Hannah who was married to Elkanah. The Bible says, "The Lord had closed her womb." (I Samuel 1: 6) Meanwhile her rival had children while Hannah waited, without even one. You may ask why did God close her womb? God was waiting for the right time to bring that child from her womb to fulfil a specific purpose on earth. When God shuts the womb, God is not saying, no you cannot have children; no, that is not His will, but he is saying that you should be patient for a while to enable Him to fulfil His purpose on earth. Hannah one day decided to draw the line. She went up to God in prayer. In her proper and beautiful passion for motherhood this desperate Hebrew mother cried unto her Lord in bitterness of soul. Hannah wept before God and prayed continuously to the Lord; she made a vow, saying, "O Lord, Almighty if you will only look upon your servant's misery and remember me and not forget your servant but give her a son, then I will give him to you Lord for all the days of his life. (I Samuel 1: 10-11)

This mother's prayer opened the door of her womb because, for the first time since she started praying, she prayed God's will for that child in her. God heard Hannah's prayers for the Bible records that "the Lord remembered her." So in the course of time Hannah conceived and gave birth to a son. (I Samuel 1: 19-20) This woman now by her promise gave God the opportunity he wanted to raise a leader for his people in a strange and difficult time.

Many women whose womb are closed may be women who want to bring children into the world to do their own will but God is saying, "that this seed that I have put in you, I want it to be used for my own glory. So mothers, what are your motives? I remember when I wanted a son. I prayed to God and asked him for a son who will be a man of prayer in His kingdom when he grows up. Within thirty days I was pregnant. Therefore our motives matter a lot. Hannah received her child as soon as her prayers lined up with the will of God for that child.

So, mothers, I advise you to do this, if you have gone for many check-ups and tests and no reason is found as to why you are not conceiving, stop running up and down - maybe God has shut your womb. No man on earth can help you. The Bible says that what He (God) shuts no man can open and what he opens no man can shut. (Isaiah 22: 22)

Even the best specialists on earth will not be able to help you, until you line yourself up for God's purpose and will to be accomplished in your life. This is what I advise you to do. Sit down at home as a couple and have a chat over a cup of tea with God - I do all the time. You may ask where will you see God? The Bible clearly tells us that God is everywhere.

> "Where can I go from your spirit? Where can I flee from your presence? If I go up to the Heavens, you are there; if I make my bed in the depths you are there; if I rise on the wings of the dawn; if I settle on the far side of the sea; even there your hand will guide me, your right hand will hold me fast." (Psalms 139: 7-10)

I just went through this Bible passage to let you know that God is omnipresent - He is everywhere, He is with us all the time. He has promised never to leave us or forsake us. You may then again ask how will you know that God is with you and is hearing you? God himself told us to come to him and we will reason together. (Isaiah 1: 18).

Imagine the God of the universe reasoning with us. But it is all true - I have done that many times. You need faith or trust to believe and know that He is there with you and once you believe that, God will speak back to you in your spirit to let you know He is with you. You may feel silly talking like that, but that is okay, as you will get used to it. The Bible says God's ear is not too dull to hear you (Isaiah 59: 1) which means that God has an ear to hear, so speak to him. If He is the one that shut that womb, He will instruct you and tell you what to do. When He instructs you, you must obey Him, for in obeying Him there is a great reward.

Examples of women in the Bible whose wombs were also shut

> Rachel's womb was shut but after much prayer God opened it. (Genesis 30: 22-23)

King Abimelech

This king took Sarah, Abraham's wife. God was not too happy about this. The Bible records in Genesis 20: 18 that: "the Lord had closed up every womb in Abimelech's household because of Abraham's wife Sarah." Even Abimelech was infertile because God had to heal him too.

Curses

A curse is a form of punishment, divine or supernatural that invokes harm or misfortune to a person in response to it. A curse can come as a result of disobedience to the Word of God or as a result of sin or family sin which children may not even be aware of. God pronounced many curses and blessings in the Bible in obedience or disobedience to His commands - for example, Deuteronomy 28 contains a list of blessings and curses for obedience or disobedience. This is an example of a curse: "You shall not worship any other God except the Lord. Cursed is any man who cast any image or cast any idol - a thing detestable to the Lord." (Deuteronomy 27: 15) In disobedience to these command, a curse on the fruit of the womb. (Deuteronomy 28: 18) Blessings also are produced on the wombs of those who serve him. (Deuteronomy 28: 4) God's Word tells us that provided His people do not bow down before other gods or worship them or follow their practices (Exodus 23: 24) "there shall be none barren [among His people]." (See also Deuteronomy 7: 13)

Lack of fruit bearing is a curse (Deuteronomy 28: 18), things like wickedness, disobedience to parents, idol worship, witchcraft, crystal ball gazers, Ouija boards, palm reading, freemasonry, etc., all bring down curses upon people. A lot of people are victims of family curses, visited on them without even knowing what their great-grandparents were involved in. Insurance companies know about those curses, that's why they ask for medical reports, etc., before giving insurance to people. They do not know these things are curses, but they surely know that certain family weaknesses are passed down from generation to generation. Infertility can run in a family as a curse.

Take a biblical example. Abraham's family problem started with Sarah. She was barren for almost ninety years; then her son Isaac married Rebekah and she was barren for twenty years (Genesis 25: 21); then Jacob married Rachel and she was also barren. (Genesis 29: 31) So we see all these men attracted to women who were barren, but Abraham was under the covenant of blessing, God had already blessed him and all these women later went on to have children, because of God's faithfulness to His Word. The curse can be destroyed from operating in one's life by taking the following steps:-

- ❖ Embrace Jesus Christ as your Lord and Saviour.
- ❖ Accept Jesus Christ and the blood he shed on the Cross for

you.
- ❖ Repent and forsake any known and unknown personal or family weakness or sin.

Not serving God

A decision not to serve God or acknowledge who he is and to reject Jesus Christ can led to infertility by bringing a curse upon such persons. God told His children that they should "worship the Lord your God and His blessing would be on your food and water and none would be barren in your land." (Exodus 23: 25-26) This shows that fruitfulness is tied up to serving God. The Bible says:

> "You have forgotten God your Saviour, you have not remembered the rock your fortress, therefore though you set out the finest plants and imported vines, yet your harvest will be nothing." (Isaiah 17: 10-11)

This passage clearly addresses those who have rejected God, even the best doctors in the world will not be able to help any man who turns his back on God. No harvest is what God promises such people; until they come back to Jesus Christ and submit to His authority, they may never conceive.

A life without prayer

A person who does not pray could find themselves held in bondage for a long time because prayer is the only thing that changes situations. If you notice, in the Bible all the couples who faced infertility were able to overcome it through prayer - Abraham prayed (Genesis 15: 1-5), Isaac prayed (Genesis 25: 21), Rachel prayed (Genesis 30: 22), Hannah prayed (I Samuel 1: 10), Manoah prayed (Judges 13: 8), Elizabeth and Zachariah prayed (Luke 1: 13); and through prayer God turned their situation around and blessed them with children. In his book, *Prayer Power*, my pastor Matthew Ashimolow called prayer, "The Christian's pilgrim staff to walk with God always. It is a mine that is full of rich supernatural minerals to be brought out, a Heaven unroughed by storm. When we are engaged in prayer, we discover the fact that it is the root, the foundation and the mother of a thousand blessings." From this quotation we can clearly see that anyone who says that they are walking with

God, and yet do not pray, are deceiving themselves. You cannot walk a fruitful walk with God without prayers. The foundation of your blessing is not laid so how can you give birth to a thousand blessings? Today I encourage you to start praying if you have not been praying. If you pray, in prayer you start to give birth to all your blessings.

What is prayer?

Personally I have found prayer to be the chain that links me to God. I have found prayer to be like the umbilical cord, the rope-like structure connecting the foetus to the placenta that supplies oxygen and nutrients from the mother's own circulation. As long as that baby is the womb, the baby remains connected to the mother through this cord for oxygen and nourishment. I have also found that as long as I remain in Christ I must stay connected to God, through the cord of prayer. Through this connection I am well nourished and cared for, well protected from all harm and danger, well-equipped for every good work.

Personally, prayer is where I live; the very breath I take every day is prayer. I have discovered prayer to be something wonderful and alive. I have no rules attached to where I must pray. I pray all the time and everywhere. I manage what quiet time I can as a mother of two little children. It is not always easy to find quiet times. But I have not allowed this to stop me praying. I pray always, before I start, I always tell the Lord to pick the prayer from the children's noise. To His glory, all these prayers are always answered. My two year old loves to pray so he always comes when I have my quiet time. He thinks it is singing time - not praying time; so no rules, we just keeping praying and God keeps answering.

My advice to you

This advice is especially for mothers with little children or those who don't have time to pray at home. Always make an effort to pray, no matter where you are, and make time to spend quiet times with God, even if you commune with God for only five or ten minutes a day. Then pray while you do other things around the house or office, quietly or in your spirit. I believe if you desire to pray the Holy Spirit will help you with a plan of prayer suitable for you. But pray always; prayer changes everything.

A family of seven brothers all under a curse of infertility

(Matthew 22: 25)

I asked the Holy Spirit to show me examples of male infertility in the Bible and this was one of them:

> Now there were seven brothers among us. The first married and died, and since he had no children, he left his wife to his brother. The same thing happened to the second and third brothers, right on down to the seventh. (Matthew 22: 25-26)

The Lord told me that this family had a curse of infertility. All men in the family were infertile. Notice the wordings carefully: "He died...he had no children." The same thing happened to all seven of them. Why? Because none of them prayed to reverse the curse. Prayer changes everything. When you pray mountains come down, situations change Prayer and praise are the Christian weapon of warfare. There is nothing on earth that cannot be conquered by praise and prayer. This family of seven brothers could not pray and they all died without leaving any issue simply because they would not pray.

Another biblical example of male infertility is found in Genesis 20: 17: "Then Abraham prayed to God, and God healed Abimelech, his wife and his slave girls so they could have children again." God had rendered Abimelech infertile because of taking another man's wife.

Emotional factors

Emotions can be blamed for some causes of infertility. The Holy Spirit has actually shown me some of the emotional factors that are likely to hinder fertility in the lives of people. Medically it is believed that excess stress can lead to impotence and reduce sperm count in men although this is difficult to quantify. It is generally thought that emotional trauma can account for ten to fifteen per cent of cases of infertility.

Worry, anxiety

All these can lead to infertility by shutting down the body's system and causing it not to function properly. During my research for this book I discovered that all the couples who faced infertility were victims of one or all of the above symptoms. God did not design our body system for worry. The Bible tells us to: "Cast all our cares on the Lord because he cares for us." He told us: "Cast all your anxiety on him because he cares for you." (I Peter 5: 7) The Lord Jesus Christ asked us this question: "Which of you by worrying can add a single hair to his life?" I want to ask you a question - how will your worrying produce that child which you desire? Many couples reading this book can testify that their worrying about this problem has not in any way helped them. The Bible says that, "A calm and undisturbed mind and heart are the life and health of the body." (Proverbs 14: 30)

The Bible says: "A glad heart makes a cheerful countenance, but by sorrow of the heart the spirit is broken. (Proverbs 15: 13) Just from these two Bible passages you can see that worrying destroys the body system. A calm and undisturbed mind and heart are the life and health of the body. So when worry sets in it starts to destroy the life of the body; it releases toxins into the body. Worry breeds more worry until one is almost going out of one's mind because of it. The Bible says that it breaks the spirit. Once a man's spirit is broken he is finished - the body becomes weak, the mind starts to play games, the body system becomes clogged up, and many organs in the body are affected.

The Holy Spirit told me that worrying and anxiety lead to infertility because the body system is not relaxed and a baby needs a relaxed atmosphere to implant itself in the womb. Please stop worrying and cast all your cares upon the Lord. God really cares for you and will surely bless you if you stop worrying and trust Him for all your needs.

Bitterness and unforgiveness

Bitterness - Many people have become infertile today because of bitterness. Bitterness is equivalent to sin for Peter said in Acts 8: 23, "for I see you are full of bitterness and captive to sin." When bitterness comes, it takes along its neighbour, sin. A bitter person always thinks his or her bitterness is justified - "Oh you don't know what he or she did to me!" Such people do not realise that bitterness will cost them more than what those people did to them. The Bible warns us thus: "See to it that no one misses the Grace of God and that no bitter root grows up to cause trouble and defile many. (Hebrews 12: 15) When a bitter root is growing many are defiled. Do you think bitterness is hindering you from conceiving? Are you bitter towards someone?

What is bitter? Bitter is distressing, galling, an expression of severe grief.

What is a root? It is the (underground) part of a flowering plant that usually anchors and supports it and absorbs and stores food; the end of a nerve near the brain and spinal cord. A bitter root is the equivalent of a severe, bitter, distressing enemy that absorbs all of the flowering part of your body.

You can see that if the root of bitterness is growing in a person it starts to spread all over the body. So how can bitterness and a baby grow together? You must choose what you want to grow in your body, either a baby or bitterness - one must give way to the other. When bitterness grows it devours many things; this includes the child that you are desiring, and the bitter root grows and replaces your child. All the organs in the human body work together to maintain our lives but if bitterness is growing in our bodies the effective working of our body organs is affected. God is asking you to forgive that person, no matter what they may have done to you. If you find it hard to forgive, ask God to help you. If you are sincere He will help you. That may be all you need to do in order to conceive.

A malicious and unrepentant heart

The Bible records the sad case of Michal, King Saul's daughter and the wife of King David, who died barren. The Bible records in II Samuel 6 the tragic story of this woman. Her husband, King David went to bring back the Ark of God from the house of Obed-Edom to the city of David, and there was rejoicing and dancing before God.

> King David, wearing a linen ephod, danced before the Lord with all His might, while he and the entire house of Israel brought up the Ark of God with shouts and sounds of trumpets. As the ark of the Lord was entering the City of David, [his wife] Michal, daughter of Saul watched from a window. And when she saw King David leaping and dancing before the Lord, she despised him in her heart. (II Samuel 6: 14-16)

> When David returned home to bless his household, Michal [his wife], daughter of Saul came out to meet him and said, "How the King of Israel has distinguished himself today, disrobing in the sight of the handmaids of his servants as any vulgar fellow would."...And Michal daughter of Saul had no

children to the day of her death. (II Samuel 6: 20, 23)

Why? She despised God and despised her husband. She had no place for God in her heart. She despised a man for worshipping God. She hated her husband, she did not reverence or cherish him one bit. She did not have a repentant heart - not even once do we read of her asking God to forgive her or asking her husband to forgive her. We do not read once about her praying for God to bless her with children like Hannah did, or Rachel or Manoah etc. All of the other women of God who were childless, prayed and the Lord later blessed them with children. Michal died barren because she hated her husband, she hated God, she was too proud to apologise and too proud to pray. In contrast we read and know that David was a man with a repentant heart. If he had offended Michal he would have repented and the Bible would have recorded it.

The Bible says God is faithful and just to forgive us for all unrighteousness, But we must pray and ask him to forgive us. If Michal had asked, God would have shown her mercy, but pride did not allow her to, therefore she died barren. So listen, women; if you are a woman who always despises your husband and other people around you, you have no place for God in your life. If you are doing all these things and have difficulty conceiving, maybe you have a lot of apologising and repenting to do. Ask your husband and those you might have hurt to forgive you and then ask God to wash and cleanse you with the blood of Jesus Christ. This may be all you need to do and before you know it you will be pregnant in Jesus' name.

Some people want to argue, "Well, I know women who beat their husbands and still have lots of children. Well, you better forget those people and settle your account with God; it could be that their sins have not caught up with them as yet, but they will later. If a woman with children beats her husband and insults him, later on in life, she will be shocked to find all those children doing the same to their spouses. She may well live to regret her ways, for you can start afresh and raise a family that will bring glory to God on earth.

When I first knew the Lord and gave my heart to him, I would see some of my friends doing certain things and I would say, "Oh, let me try doing this too," and the Lord would clearly warn me, saying: "Vero do not try it, for you will not get away with it." The voice of the Lord helped to restrain me because I knew I could not get away with doing the same things that others were doing. God deals with us individually, one person may do something and keep getting away with it, while another could try it and face dire consequences. So let us remain broken and repentant so that God's blessing may continue to flow in our life - let us not be like Michal.

The blessing of a repentant heart - Sarah

The Bible records in Genesis 11: 30 that Sarah, Abraham's wife was barren and bore him no children. Then God said to Abram: "I will make you into a great nation and will bless you. (Genesis 12: 2) After God had spoken and revealed His will to this couple, Sarah took no heed and she quickly devised her own plans. She told Abraham to sleep with her maid to enable her to build a family. Abraham agreed to this plan and went to be with Sarah's maid, Hagar, and she conceived. Abraham did not take a stand on the Word that God spoke to him.

When Hagar conceived that is when the real war began in Abraham's house. In Genesis 16 we read of fighting and quarrelling between Sarah, Hagar and Abraham himself. Talking about Sarah, we read of a woman who laughed when God told her He would bless her and make her a mother but later she was quick to admit that the joke was on her. (Genesis 18: 12, 15)

We read of a woman who agreed time and again to go with other men at the suggestion of her husband. (Genesis 12: 11-15, 20: 1-3) We read of a woman who did not think twice before giving another woman to her husband and we read of a husband who never gave a thought to the fact that his wife could be raped or sexually abused. We read of a couple, especially of a woman, who did not take the promise of God seriously. We read of a woman who loved fighting. We read in Genesis what Sarah finally did to Hagar after Isaac was born. One day the son of the slave woman mocked Isaac (his name was Ishmael), the offspring of a failure of faith. It was now necessary for Hagar and Ishmael to be sent away for they could not have a part in the purpose of God, which God had planned to achieve through His chosen people.

We read in the Bible how Sarah handled this issue, she said to Abraham: "Get rid of that slave woman and her son for that slave woman will never share in the inheritance with my son." (Genesis 21: 10) This was the same woman on whom Sarah had built her hopes of raising a family. She did not care any more. Can you imagine the scene that day in Abraham's house as Sarah made sure she got her way? The Bible records that this matter distressed Abraham because it concerned his son, Ishmael. (Genesis 20: 11) I am sure Abraham was ready to deal severely with Sarah that day; after all she was the one who persuaded him to sleep with Hagar. She was the one who created the terrible situation in the house, but thank God for His mercy. That day God intervened in that family to bring peace back to the home. God said to Abraham: "Do not be distressed about the boy and your maidservant. Listen to whatever Sarah tells you." (Genesis 21: 11-12) So Abraham listened to God, and did what Sarah said, and sent Hagar and Ishmael away.

Whilst all this was going on, God was working in the life of Sarah and Abraham. It took many years but the Bible says, "God changes us from glory to glory." At times it looks slow but God takes His time to accomplish His purpose in our lives. God could easily have given Sarah a child, when he gave Hagar Ishmael, but I have since learnt that God cannot be blackmailed or bullied into doing anything. God had to accomplish His perfect will in Sarah's life. The Bible records that Sarah obeyed Abraham and called him her master. She changed into a new woman, and she even obeyed her husband and submitted to him. Thus God blessed her and also said to us women that we will be Sarah's daughters, if we do what is right and do not give way to fear. (I Peter 3: 6) Sarah was blessed by God and she lived in peace and brought Isaac up in a godly home without quarrelling and fighting; God had finally finished His perfect work in her life. I want to advise husbands and wives, if they are still playing cat and mouse like Abraham and Sarah, that they might be the ones delaying their child from coming. God may just be waiting for them to put their houses in order and to create an atmosphere conducive for those special children he wants to give to them. He may not want such a child to be born into a household where the child will witness his parents fighting and wrestling with each other. Isaac was a special child, God wanted him to be born into a peaceful and godly home. Your forthcoming baby may be the same, so get your home in order.

Many people will say, "Well I know a lot of couples who fight every day and yet they have children." Please, I advise you to forget those people; if they are fighting and have children, this is not your portion. Therefore do not concern yourself about them - for every man will reap what he sows. I cannot emphasise enough that both of you must make a commitment to God to help you to change and bring peace into your home, in Jesus' name, Amen.

Isaac - a blessed man

God's initial preparation for the coming of Isaac into Abraham's home paid off. Reading through the Bible, he is one of the few men who really loved his wife. The Bible records that Isaac brought her into the tent of his mother, Sarah, and married Rebekah. So she became his wife, and he loved her. (Genesis 24: 67)

After this marriage, Rebekah did not get pregnant for almost twenty years - what did Isaac do? Did he marry another woman, have concubines? The answer is no. The Bible records that Isaac prayed to the Lord on behalf of his wife because she was barren.

The Lord answered his prayer and his wife became pregnant. (Genesis 25: 20-21) What a man! Mothers, I pray that you will make your home a place of peace and love where you can raise up great husbands like Isaac, men who will pray for their wives in both difficult and good times.

Impatience

One of the causes of Infertility is impatience. While researching for this book, I discovered that a lot of couples were unwilling to try for any period of time before embarking on a fertility treatment. Their doctors may say to them, "Wait a little longer, try for some time first," but they, being unwilling to wait a little longer, embark and pay thousands of pounds for fertility treatments that end up not working. They fail to achieve a conception, lose a lot of money and come back home broken and battered, both physically and emotionally. The tampering with the body, especially a woman's body, in most cases ends up creating problems that were not in existence before the treatment was embarked upon. One of the things I have learnt to cultivate whilst walking with the Lord is patience. No human being can walk a fruitful walk with God, without patience. The Bible clearly tells us that there is a waiting time. "Then those that wait upon the Lord ,shall renew their strength, they shall mount up with wings as Eagles, they shall run and not be weary. They shall walk and not faint." (Isaiah 40: 31)

While you wait on God, He will renew your strength, He will encourage you and strengthen you, He will give you an assurance that everything is under His control. Humble yourself, therefore under God's mighty hand that He may lift you up in due time. (I Peter 5: 6) There is a due time with God and when the time is due nothing will stop that child from being born in Jesus' name.

Wickedness

This is another cause of infertility among so many today. In Deuteronomy 27, there are many curses and all of them involve one form of wickedness or another. One example is this: "Cursed is the man who withholds justice from the alien, the fatherless or the widow." (Deuteronomy 27: 19) The Bible says in Proverbs 3: 33: "The Lord's curse is on the house of the wicked, but he blesses the home of the righteous. One of these curses is the curse of the fruit of the womb (Deuteronomy 28: 18). "The way of the wicked is like deep darkness; they do not know what makes them stumble. (Proverbs 4: 19)

From this passage of scripture we can see that the wicked man knows he is falling, but he does not know what makes him stumble and fall. The Bible says the house of the wicked will be destroyed, but the tent of the upright will flourish. (Proverbs 14: 11)

"House of the wicked" includes their seed, their children, their womb, eggs, sperm and everything that pertains to them, for the sacrifice of the wicked is detestable to the Lord. In Hosea 9 God spoke about the penalty of wickedness. "Because of their wickedness in Gilgai I hated them, Because of their sinful deeds. I will drive them out of my house. Their root is withered, they yield no fruit." (Hosea 9: 15-16, Proverbs 15: 8) From these Bible passages you can see there is no hope for a wicked man until he turns from his wicked ways back to God. We now go to the Bible to read about infertility due to wickedness.

This story is found in Genesis 38 about Judah, his sons and Tamar, their wife. It is a case of male infertility due to wickedness. Judah had two sons named Er and Onan. "One day Judah took a wife for his eldest son; her name was Tamar. Er, Judah's first-born, was wicked in the sight of God, so the Lord put him to death. Then Judah said to Onan his second son, 'Marry your brother's widow, live with her and raise offspring for your brother.' So whenever he lay with his brother's widow, he spilled his semen on the ground to keep him from producing offspring for his brother. What he did was wicked in the Lord's sight so he put him to death also." We see two brothers whose wickedness robbed them of their seed. They used their own wickedness on themselves. They died without having any children, for the Word of God says, "both were wicked men". No wonder the Bible says, "the house of the wicked will be destroyed." (Proverbs 14: 11)

Note here that Tamar was not infertile - she was a good woman who married evil men. She was sent away with a deceptive promise by her father-in-law, back to her own family for many years, and was forgotten by the family she married into. One day she heard that her father-in-law was passing by her village on his way to shear his sheep. She disguised herself and went out and her father-in-law thought she was a prostitute and slept with her. That same day she became pregnant. The Bible says, "about three months later Judah was told, your daughter-in-law, Tamar, is guilty of prostitution and as a result is pregnant." Judah said: "Bring her out and burn her to death." Then she bought out the seal and cord which her wicked father-in-law had used to pay her for sex on that day, thinking she was a prostitute. She said, "I am pregnant by the man who owns these. See if you recognise them." Then Judah recognised them and said, "She is more righteous than I am." From this story we learn of Judah's sons who were wicked men; both died childless because of wickedness. Er died without children, Onan had seed in him but he wasted his semen rather than produce children with it. What a shame. The Bible says that, "those who plough evil and those who sow trouble reap it." (Job 4: 8) Therefore married couples who are finding it difficult to conceive need to check themselves for any form of wickedness as this could be the reason for their not having children at this present moment. You must examine yourself and repent of your wickedness. You say, "Is there hope for me?" "Yes, God says, 'If you return to him, he will return to you.'" (Zachariah 1: 3) God says, "I will restore you to health and heal all your wounds." (Isaiah 30: 26) Turning away from wickedness brings you back to God's blessing.

God is merciful; once you repent he throws away all the wicked acts you have done and puts the righteousness of Christ upon you. You become a new person in Christ.

Not faithful in tithes

One other cause of infertility is not bringing your tithes into the house of God. What are tithes? A tithe is literally ten per cent of your gross income. In the Old Testament God asked His people: "Will a man rob God or defraud me? But you say, "In what way do we rob and defraud you?" The answer is that you have withheld your tithes and offerings. You are cursed with a curse for you are robbing me, "even this whole nation." "Bring all the tithes [the whole tenth of your income] into the store house, that there may be food in my house and test me in this," says the Lord of Host, "and see if I will not open the windows of Heaven for you and pour out such a blessing that you shall not have room enough to receive it. I will prevent pests (disease, *sickness*) from devouring your crops; neither shall your vine drop its fruit before the time in the field (miscarriage, *sickness*), says the Lord of host and all nations shall call you happy and blessed for yours shall be a delightful land," says the Lord Almighty. (Malachi 3: 8-12) There is a level of blessing attached to faithfulness in tithing. The Heavens are open to those who give and God's protection is upon them and their family. For a person who brings in their tithe, the blessing written above is upon them, but for those people who refuse to bring their tithes into the house of God, the devourer is let loose upon their life. Miscarriages, still births are just some of the curses upon those who do not tithe. You may say well that this was in the Old Testament. No, not by any means; our Lord Jesus Christ in the New Testament mentioned tithes - in Matthew 25: 23, in Luke 18: 12. In Hebrews 7: 6 tithing was mentioned, confirming that even in our current generation tithing must continue. When you bring you tithe into the church or towards the work of God, it helps to keep the Gospel going, and it helps to aid less privileged people. But when you hoard what is meant for the glory of God you cheat only yourself out of God's blessing. You may say well "many people don't tithes yet they are blessed with healthy childern" I have since learnt that in every situation in life I must leave other people alone and obey the Word of God. The Bible command us to tithes and that is what we must do.

My personal experience

Because of my faithfulness to tithing, God's protection has been upon my home and my children. Three times the courts have sent bailiffs to come and take my house, but they have not succeeded because God's protection is on my home. Sickness is far from my home and my children, because of God's protection. I have never lacked anything, even what I will bless others with. God has continued to be faithful to me.

When the teachers at my daughter's school tried to put a label on my daughter, saying that she needed a "special school" in order to learn to speak, God immediately turned their report into foolishness. Within the term I received a letter from the same teacher telling me my daughter was the best girl in the school. Why? - because of my faithfulness in giving tithes and offering. I have received so many other benefits because of my tithing which I will share with you in my other books. I will encourage you to start tithing faithfully from now on.

If you are not sure about tithing, talk to God about this and he himself will minister to you concerning the issue of tithing. He will direct you in

His wisdom about what you should do. God Bless You.

Sexual immorality

The Bible clearly warns us to keep away from sexual immorality, impurity and lust, which bring down the wrath of God. (Colossians 3: 5-6) Having many different partners usually leads to the infliction of such venereal diseases as gonorrhoea and chlamydia. They lead to inflammation and, if not treated early, could give rise to blockages, leading to infertility.

A promiscuous lifestyle could later on in life result in damage to the womb, blockage of the Fallopian tubes or even result in the woman becoming sterile. In the Bible, such acts as sleeping with one's daughter, sister, etc., carried a curse upon it. (Deuteronomy 27: 22) In the world today, many people do all these things and get away with it, but for some, they may not be so lucky, so if you find yourself caught up in any of these things, you may need to repent and tell God you are sorry and He will forgive you. This may be all you need to do to conceive.

Biblical examples of sexual immorality - Genesis 20

Abraham and Abimelech

Infertility due to sexual immorality - in Genesis 20 we read of Abraham and Abimelech. Abraham had left the south country of Negeb and arrived in Gerar. Here he told his wife to lie and to say that she was his sister, so Sarah lied and King Abimelech sent for Sarah and took her. Here was a king with so many wives, yet sexual immorality had bound him. He could not resist a beautiful woman but the Bible records, "God came to Abimelech in a dream by night and said, 'Behold you are dead because of the woman whom you have taken as your own, for she is another man's wife.'" (Genesis 20: 3) Abimelech tried to explain to God that he was innocent in this matter, but God said to him, "Yes, I know you did this with a clear conscience, and so I spared you from sinning against me. That is why I did not let you touch her. (Genesis 20: 6) God commanded the king to return Sarah to Abraham. When the king returned her to Abraham, Abraham prayed to God and God healed Abimelech and his wife and his female slaves and they bore children, for the Lord had closed tightly the wombs of all Abimelech's household, because of Sarah, Abraham's wife. (Genesis 20: 17-18)

Many will say, "Well! Everyone is sleeping with everyone and getting away with it." That's fine but for some people it may not be that easy.

If you are involved in sexual immorality, I will advise you to turn away from it and ask God to forgive you and heal you. God is faithful and just and will forgive you - in Jesus' name. Other biblical examples are:

> If a man sleeps with his aunt, he has dishonoured his uncle. They will be held responsible. They will die childless.
>
> If a man marries his brother's wife, it is an act of impurity; he has dishonoured his brother. They will be childless. (Found in Leviticus 20: 20 -21)

King David (2 Samuel 11)

One of the greatest men who lived on earth did not escape the curse of sexual immorality. The Bible records that in the spring, at the time when kings go to war, David sent off his fighting men and stayed at home. One evening David got up from his bed and walked around on the roof. He saw a beautiful woman bathing and David sent for her. She came to him and he slept with her. Then she went back home. The woman conceived and sent word to David, saying, "I am pregnant."

This woman was Bathsheba. She was a married woman, and her husband was among the fighting men David sent off to war. When David discovered this woman was pregnant, he sent for her husband to come back home from war so that he would go home and make love to his wife thus passing off the pregnancy to this man. When Uriah, Bathsheba's husband, came, David urged him to go home and wash his feet. Uriah said to David, "The ark and Israel and Judah are staying in the tents, and my master Joab and my Lord's men are camped in the open fields. How could I go to my house to eat and drink and lie with my wife? As surely as the Lord lives I will not do such a thing. This man was a godly man. This man loved and revered God. He loved God and respected the king. His decision not to go home and sleep with his wife cost him his life, for when he went back to war the next day, King David sent him with a letter which carried his death sentence. He was put in the place where the battle was fiercest and was killed. David sent for his wife and married her.

God's judgement

The first thing that God told the king was, "out of your own household, I am going to bring calamity upon you. Before your eyes I will take your wives and give them to one who is close to you, and he will lie with your wives in broad daylight."

The second judgement was that the child conceived through that act of sexual immorality died. Then David comforted his wife Bathsheba and went to her and lay with her. She gave birth to a son and they named him Solomon. The Lord loved him. (II Samuel 12: 11, 24)

Solomon

Solomon was a son born to David through this marriage. He was blessed and loved by God, He ended up as the wisest man that ever lived. He was one of the richest men who ever lived and he had tasted just about everything life had to offer- He had beautiful women in his life, He was wise, lived a luxurious life style and had everything life had to offer at his disposal. He still ended up marrying seven hundred wives of royal birth and three hundred concubines. (I Kings 11: 3) So watch out for sexual immorality. If you escape infertility, your children could end up with sexual problems too much for them to handle and may not know it was your immoral behaviour that has been passed on to them.

At the end of all his sexual adventures I would like to leave you with a statement made by this great man. He said, "All is meaningless, meaningless, chasing after wind." (Ecclesiastes 1: 2) After sampling everything life had to offer this great man had only one advice to give to us - it proved meaningless. So, if you are wise, listen to the words of the most sexually immoral man that ever lived. It was not worth it.

Chapter Sixteen

More Questions: What Of Infertility Among Christians?

During my research for this book I discovered that infertility affects as many Christians as non-Christians. I also discovered that most Christians had excuses as to why they were infertile, statements like, "God is using it to make us love him better", "serve him better", "teach us a lesson", "does not hear my prayer", were common statements made by God's people. Today under the clear leadership of the Holy Spirit I have decided to answer some of the major questions asked on this issue. The first statement I am going to make is this: infertility among Christians can be attributed to one reason and that is *not knowing God's will and purpose!*

God himself said this in Hosea 4: 6 "my people are destroyed for lack of knowledge;" God did not attribute destruction of our lives and lack to the devil or infertility, he attributed it to lack of knowledge. When we lack knowledge of the will and purpose of God for our lives, then the consequences are great. From the day God created man on the face of the earth, His will and purpose was made clear: "Be fruitful and increase in number, fill the earth and subdue it." (Genesis 1: 28) When God took His people out of the land of Egypt, God again told them: "I love you and will bless you and increase your numbers. I will bless the fruit of your womb. You will be blessed more than any other people; none of your men or women will be childless." (Deuteronomy 7: 13-14)

In Deuteronomy 28: 4 God again confirms His blessing on His people: "the fruit of your womb will be blessed." Here we see God's desire and will for His people; the Christians - those who believe in Christ Jesus - God himself meets all their needs, supplies all their demands. Everything related to a Christian is to bear a mark of prosperity and success. God again speaks in Malachi 2: 5. "My covenant with him was a covenant of life and peace..." That is for every Christian, not only spiritual but physical life; His covenant with His people is one of life, not death - for a man or woman who believes in Him.

There is no way whatsoever that a Christian who believes these promises from God's Word can remain sick or infertile, because God's Word cannot fail. If God said, "...none of those who serve him will be barren," then that's exactly what it means: none means none to God. In Christ Jesus, God's promise to all Christians is fruitfulness - children - for the Bible says: "if a man remains in me and I in him, he will bear much fruit." (John 15: 5)

As long as you belong to Christ, God's promise to you is to have children.

My own personal experience of ignorance of God's word

In August 1992. I gave my heart to the Lord. Soon after this experience, burglars started coming into my home. Several times they came in and stole valuable things. Finally I cried out to the Lord to ask why this was happening to me. He then answered me by saying I was not releasing the ministry angels. Let's look at Hebrews 1: 14.

Are not all angels ministering spirits sent to serve those who will inherit salvation?

Those who will inherit salvation? The ministering angels are here to serve us but if you have someone sent to serve you what must you do? You must give them specific instructions as to what you want them to do. The Lord told me that it was ignorance of His Word that caused me to lose all those things through a thief. After that day I started instructing my ministering angels every day as to what I wanted them to do. Until the time of writing this it has been three years and no thief has ever come near my home. Glory be to God. His Word is true, it can never fail.

God created man to multiply and increase and subdue the earth. God gave man the power to have control over every situation in the earth. Man is to use the power of God's Word to change whatever situation he does not like.

Question

Does God use infertility to make us love him more and serve him better?

This is probably one of the greatest deception of that enemy of man, Satan.

If he can get the Christians to believe this lie, soon we will have no more witness.

What will happen if Christians decide not to have children in order to serve God better? What would have happened if after God created Adam and Eve they decided not to obey God's command to multiply and fill the earth so that they can love *and serve God* better? The earth would have remained empty and you and I would never have been born. It is God's perfect will, His desire for every Christian to have children. Why?

To have a witness to the world

Christians must have children who will be witness to the world, bringing the gospel to the ends of the earth. If God denies the Christians children, soon no one would be left to carry God's message to the ends of the earth.

His blessings are tied up in our children

God himself is our Heavenly Father and also the Father of our Lord Jesus Christ; the Bible says that God so loved the world that he gave His only begotten son. Why? God knew the importance of children. When mankind sank into sin, God needed someone to help him restore mankind to him. God himself needed help and His son was there to help. No one knows more about the importance of children in our life than God himself.

For these are God's command to the children of Israel, His children.

> "These commands that I give you today are to be upon your hearts Impress them on your children. Talk about them when you sit at home and when you walk along the road, when you lie down and when you get up." (Deuteronomy 6: 6-7)

We can clearly see that God's desire is to bless us with children who we will teach His ways to and that they in turn should teach their own children. God's blessing is meant to rest upon a thousand generations of those who love and fear him. (Deuteronomy 5: 10)

Abraham had a promise from God, that promise was a promise

which involved the blessing of children.

> "I will bless her [Sarah] and will surely give you a son by her. I will bless her so that she will be the mother of nations; kings of people will come from her." (Genesis 17: 16)

When King David who also walked with God wanted to build God a house, (temple) God said to him, "...your son whom I will put on the throne in your place will build the temple for my name." (I Kings 5: 5)

David was a man who loved God and served God, yet God blessed him with children. God had plans for David as well as His son. All God's plans are tied up with our children and loving and serving Him is also part of His plan. Having children does not stop us from serving God or loving Him. God himself said: "It is not good for man to be alone - I will make him a helper suitable for him. (Genesis 2: 18)

This God did by taking the ribs of the man and forming a woman for him. (Genesis 2: 21) Even this woman was not enough. God also commanded them to multiply and fill the earth. God loved Adam and Eve, he wanted them to serve Him, for the Bible records that "he came in the cool of the evening to the garden..." in order to be in fellowship with them. (Genesis 3: 8)

Having children does not in any way hinder one from serving God. Rather it enhances our service to God. The decision to serve God and not have children must be a personal decision for you, from your own heart (of your own will), because that is not God's will. If you feel not having children will make you serve God better, then that is what you should say, but please don't say it is God who is denying you children to enable you to serve Him better. That contradicts the Bible and the nature of God.

Who said: "I'm the Lord, I change not."? (Malachi 3: 6) The God who in Genesis said, "...everything produces after its kind and the seed is in itself." So God has already put the seed in you to bring forth children when you were born. There is no way that He will deny you that which He has promised you. Has the God who said, "None in my house shall be barren," changed His mind? *No* - He remains true and faithful to the end, No child of God will be denied his inheritance if he goes for it. For the Bible says: "Sons are a heritage from the Lord, children a reward from him. (Psalms 127: 3)

Question

"Before I became a Christian I had one (or more) abortions, which led to many medical complication in my reproductive organs. Now that I am a Christian, will I be able to have children? What is my position spiritually on this issue?

Before we proceed with this question we must first find out the meaning of the word abortion. What is abortion? Abortion is the premature termination of a pregnancy by taking a foetus from its mother's womb. Abortion can be induced or may be spontaneous.

Medically induced abortion: this is where a woman consents to a doctor terminating the life of her unborn child. It may be medically advised, as in cases where doctors feel conditions exist that could endanger the life of the mother or child. Women who accidentally become pregnant and do not want to bring such a child into the world might also choose to have such babies aborted. Abortion is very common among the young women of our generation due to sexual promiscuity.

Spontaneous abortion

This is where a woman who is pregnant loses or miscarries the baby. Many reason are attributed to the cause of this.

The abortion I will be discussing here is induced abortion - where a woman deliberately decides to terminate the life of the child in her womb. The first statement I will make here is that, "Abortion is a heinous crime against God." Yes, each time a life is brutally taken away, it is a crime against God. For the Bible clearly says: " ***Thou shall not kill***." (Exodus 20: 13)

This question came up because I discovered that a lot of women in the church were worried because the abortion they had had before becoming Christians still haunted them. They also felt a sense of guilt about it. It is right to feel guilt about abortion because abortion itself is murder. Where a woman deliberately takes the life of her unborn offspring that is murder. It is a fact that criminal abortions usually performed by quack doctors in haste in ill-equipped clinics are many times more dangerous to the mother than normal childbirth. It is the general testimony of legitimate physicians that even though the mother survives the shock of this terrible outrage against God and nature, she is often doomed to a life of suffering and misery - physically, mentally and morally. Hence the guilt experienced by so many of my sisters in the Lord, who have had one or more abortions.

Today I want to bring you the good news that, while abortion is wrong and a sin against God, by the blood of Jesus Christ, which He shed on the Cross, that abortion is dealt with. The power of the blood of Jesus removed all that separated you from God. That same blood that Jesus shed for you has dealt with all your sins, and you are perfected by His blood. God does not remember your sins (abortions), not one of them, for the Bible declares what the Lord says: "...for I will forgive their wickedness and will remember their sins no more." (Jeremiah 31: 34) Every sin is forgotten by the blood of Jesus. Every sin has been washed away and this gives you unlimited access to the very throne room of God.

For the Bible says: "Now in Christ Jesus, you, who once were far away, have been brought near through the blood of Christ." (Ephesians 2: 13) The blood of Jesus has restored your relationship and fellowship with God. You stand before God as a righteous person; the Bible says that the blood that the sinless Son of God shed for you makes you perfect.

Today I want to encourage you, my beautiful sisters, to let go. At times it is more difficult for us to forgive ourselves because God has already forgiven us. Forgive yourself and put that guilt under the blood of Jesus Christ and serve God with peace of mind. For who the Lord shall set free is free indeed. (I shall write a book on abortion in the future.)

Secondly now that you are a Christian you are now in the family of God, and the Bible declares all things are yours. In the Family of God, your Father is the Father who will never give His child a stone for bread. You have a Father who loves you with an everlasting love, a Father who gave His best in Jesus Christ to redeem you from sin and death. You are a blessed woman; in the family of God no one shall be childless.

I want you to know today that If you will forgive yourself and ask God to heal or bless you with children, He will surely bless you. For the Bible says that He who ask receives. Remember God has forgiven you and He loves you. God bless you.

Question

What of those who refuse to have children?

Those who make this decision not to have children as a result of childhood experiences such as incest, rape, multiple abortion, may do so because all these experiences might have planted fear in their hearts.

The first thing I want us to get clear is that having children is a blessing from God. For God's command to man in Genesis was: "Be fruitful and multiply and replenish the earth." (Genesis 1: 28)

Those who are coming from such family background often make inner vows, such as: "I will never have children in my life-time. I will never bring children into the world to suffer what I suffered in my childhood." Many people become so afraid of a repetition of that which happened to them happening again to their children that they make decisions not to have children at all.

Today I bring you the good news that Jesus loves you and cares for you; He wants you to know that He is more than able to protect you and put right anything that is wrong in your life. Your decision not to have children through fears of the past is wrong. If you are a Christian and serving God, the blood of Jesus is able to heal you and restore you. The same blood is enough to protect any child or children you may bring into the world. The blood of Jesus is enough to destroy every curse that might have come as a result of the abuse you underwent as a child.

God has told us in His Word not to be afraid of anything. Time and time again he tells us: "Do not fear." Why? Because He has not given us the Spirit of fear. God wants us to be bold and strong and full of His love. He wants you to deal with all these childhood experiences that may still be a hindrance to your life. (2 Timothy 1: 7) He says He has not given you the spirit of fear but of love and a sound mind.

This is what I will advise you to do:

- ❖ Come to God by faith.
- ❖ Tell God all your hurts and fears.
- ❖ Ask Him to help you forget all those bad experience and to heal you and to forgive you, as well as all those who hurt you in the past.
- ❖ Ask Him to bless you with children; tell Him you believe He is able to protect your children from all the nasty experience you went through.
- ❖ Believe He has done it. Keep praising him for it. God Bless You.

Now make a confession:

Father in Jesus' name I bless you. I thank you that you are my Father and that you love me so much. I made inner vows when I was a child that I will never have children beacause of all the pain and abuse I went through as a child. Father I have read your Word and I belive it to be true. I ask you in the name of Jesus' to heal me today of those hidden wound. I ask you to forgive me and to forgive all those people that have hurt me. Thank you Father for rebuilding the old waste-places of my life, I'm like a green pine tree; my fruitfulness comes from You.(Hosea 14:8).

All that the canker worm have eaten the Father is now restoring to me. The Father is like the dew to me, He makes me blossom like a lily. Like a cedar of Lebanon. His splendour is over me like an olive tree; His fragrance around me is like the cedar of Lebanon. I flourish like corn, I blossom like a vine, and His glory overflows in my life. (Hosea 14:7).

Question

What of infertility treatments among Christians?

Infertility simply means that a couple have been trying to conceive for a year or more without result. The issue of infertility treatment now comes up where a couple decides to seek help medically in an attempt to conceive. In doing this, a lot of test, medicines, surgical treatment and test tubes will be involved. A lot of money will also be involved and your strength and emotions will be taxed. Infertility is one area which the doctors will admit that they know very little of. Because of lack of light in this area, most of the time the cause of infertility cannot consequently be detected. Medically very little can be done. The reason for this is clear, as the Bible says: "the secret things belong to the Lord our God, but the things revealed belong to us and our children forever, that we may follow all the words of this law." (Deuteronomy 29: 29) The second thing is that the Word of God says in Ecclesiastes 11: 5 - that, " As you know not the path of the wind, or how the body is formed in a mother's womb, so you cannot understand the work of God, the maker of all things. The area of fertility is a secret thing that belongs to God." That's why doctors cannot understand the issue of infertility - because it is a secret thing that belongs to God. Man has his part to play ,but there are areas no one should touch.

Infertility treatment is one of the most distressing, disruptive experiences you can ever go through. Recently I prayed for a lady who had undergone infertility treatment without success; she told me: "I went through so much pain I was afraid I was going to die." Anybody who has undergone these treatments will tell you it was no joking matter. I personally believe God did not intend us to go through so much pain; that's why Christ bore all our pain on the Cross, I am sure it saddens God to see us go through this amount of pain over having children.

For the Christian couple, I guess the decision for them to undertake infertility treatment will be a hard one. There are so many treatments available today; the Christian couple will have to make a choice as to how far they are willing to go and what they are willing to try in order to conceive. Most of the treatments available are in total contradiction of the Word of God. How far you go and what you decide to do will be a choice you make here on earth and for which you may one day have to answer to God. The Bible clearly tell us God's will and promise to those who serve him. God told us in the Bible that, "none in his house will be barren." (Deuteronomy 7: 14) God also promised that He would engender a difference between those who serve him and those who don't. (Exodus 33: 16-17) So, if the people in the world are doing all this stuff and the children of God are right behind them, where is the difference which our God promised us? Either God is lying or we are totally lost, but because we all know God can never lie it means we, His children, have lost ourselves somewhere. It Is time for the children of God to wake up and take their place on the earth which God has allotted to them. Moses the servant of God knew a difference must exist between those who serve God and those who don't serve him. God told us in the Bible that, "none in his house will be barren." (Exodus 7: 14) God also promised that He will make a difference between those who serve him and those who don't. (Exodus 33: 17) If the people in the world are involved in all those treatments, the children of God who have accepted Jesus as Lord and Saviour, should be able to look up to God from where their help comes from. They should be able to advise the world that the answer is not in more embryo research, but in the Word of God. The Bible tells us not to be afraid of anything including infertility because our God will fight for us. (Deuteronomy 3: 22)

Our Lord Jesus Christ told us, "I have come into the world as a light, so that no-one who believes in me should stay in darkness." (John 12: 46)

For every child of God who knows Christ for themselves the promise is Light. God promises you Light so the darkness of infertility is not big enough to overcome you. Why then will you who have the Light start running to people who clearly admits to you that they have no light in the area of infertility? Why are you, a child of Light, running to the one who clearly admits to you that what he is doing is by trial and error, that it may succeed or fail? The Bible says, "Men cry out under a load of oppression, they plead for relief from the arm of the powerful. But no-one says, 'Where is God, my maker?'" (Job 35: 9-10) Most of the time when trouble comes who is the first person you run to? The Bible clearly answers this question for us. We run to powerful men like doctors, etc., to seek relief. We only come back to seek the face of God when all else has failed, when the arm of flesh has failed us.

You must decide what you want to do and then submit your decison to the Lord who the Bible calls, "the Lord who sent His Word and healed you." The Bible commands us to do this: "Come out from among them and be separate." (2 Corinthians 6: 17)

Let's take a Biblical example of a person who faced an illness and did not seek God.

King Asa

The Bible says that Asa's heart was fully committed to the Lord all his life.

Asa was a Christian. (2 Chronicles 15: 17)

> In the thirty-ninth year of his reign Asa was afflicted with a disease in his feet. Though his disease was severe, even in his illness **he did not seek help from the Lord but only from the physicians.** Then in the forty-first year of his reign Asa died and rested with his fathers. (2 Chronicles 16: 12-13)

One can clearly see that God was not pleased with Asa for seeking the help of man when God had promised "to be his healer". (Psalms 107: 20) Many Christian couples desiring or taking infertility treatment have not spent enough time mediating in the promises of God concerning having children, instead of seeking the face of God first, they are now relying on the physician. God uses doctors to heal and bless His people. He uses them to heal and he also uses divine healing but His primary desire is that we come to Him first, that we acknowledge him first as our healer. We should be able to say: "Father, in whatever way my healing comes, I know it comes from you. You are the God who heals me. Whatever you direct me to do, that I will do. You are the one I look up to." The point I am making here is that in all sickness, we must first seek the face of God before going to anyone else - especially in the area of infertility where the doctors have limited light. When we hand everything over to God, He will direct you to a hospital or clinic, if he wants you to go to one, He Himself will be in the doctor or nurse who will be dealing with you. He will instruct them as how best to help you. I would love to advise you that in whatever situation you find yourself try to acknowledge God first.

I am not putting down the work of doctors because they do great work. The point I am making here is that no matter what happens our hope must be built on the Word of God and not on human beings. If we do that, God's blessing flows into our lives. God's Word says to us: "Woe to those who go down to Egypt for help, who rely on horses, who trust in the multitude of their chariots and in the great strength of their horsemen, but do not look to the Holy one of Israel, or seek help from the Lord." (Isaiah 31: 1)

I want to leave you with these promises from the Bible, from the mouth of God - "You will be blessed more than any other people: none of your men or women will be childless." (Deuteronomy 7: 14)

Moses, the servant of God, asked God this question: "What else will distinguish me and my people from all the people on the face of the earth?" And the Lord said to Moses: "I will do the very thing you have asked, because I am pleased with you and I know you by name." (Exodus 33: 16-17) Moses, the servant of God, asked God to distinguish between those who didn't serve God and those who were God's people. God agreed with what Moses had asked and did just that.

The Bible says in Isaiah 31: 2: "He [God] does not take back his words." Has God changed? If you say no to this question, then you must also believe that His promise is sure and cannot fail. Below I answer two questions on the various treatments undertaken at the infertility clinics.

What about *in vitro* fertilisation and embryo freezing?

In vitro fertilisation is a method of treating infertility in which an egg is surgically removed from the ovary and fertilised outside the body. *In vitro* means "in glass". This method of treatment is undertaken when the woman's Fallopian tubes are permanently blocked or absent, where the man's sperm count is low or where there are antibodies in the woman's cervical mucus which kill the sperm.

A woman undergoing this treatment will normally be given fertility drugs during the first eight days of her menstrual cycle; this is to stimulate her eggs to ripen. After some days the woman will go through a series of ultra sound scans to monitor the ripening of the eggs in her ovaries. Immediately or before ovulation (which may be induced by drugs), ripe eggs are remove by laparoscopy or by ultra sound-guided-needle-aspiration through the vagina or abdomen. The eggs are mixed with the man's sperm in a dish which is then put in an incubator. Then the eggs are examined to see if they have been fertilised and have started to develop into embryos. Usually at the two or four cells stage, they are placed in the woman's uterus through the vagina.

Recent research shows that half or more of all eggs have abnormal chromosomes and cannot develop into normal embryos after fertilisation. The eggs begins to divide but the pregnancy miscarries.

Freezing embryos (cryopreservation)

At the temperature of liquid nitrogen, -196° C, biological materials do not deteriorate. Once an embryo is placed in a glass tube and cooled to this temperature, it can theoretically be held almost indefinitely.

When used

Quite often more than three eggs are fertilised in a single IVF cycle but legally only three can be implanted at once. Many clinics now have the facilities for freezing the remaining embryo.

These methods are used:
A) When couples wish to keep them so that they can be used in the future.
B) Where embryos are produced but the mother reacts to the drug treatment in such a way that they cannot be immediately placed in her womb.

It is a fact that the process of freezing may in itself cause damage so that either the embryo may not grow properly or possibly the resulting child may experience some problems when he or she grows up to be an adult.

What the Bible says

The issue of IVF and embryo freezing is a very delicate one. A lot of people will argue and say, "Well, that was the only option left for me, to be able to have children." There are many thing we do that are the only options left for us, and yet as children of God those things may be good, but they may not be God's perfect Will for us.

In the beginning of creation, God created every living thing and put it in its natural environment. God said:

> "...let birds fly above the earth across the expanse of the sky." So God created the great creatures of the sea and every living and moving thing with which the water teems, according to their kinds, and every winged bird according to its kind...God blessed them and said, "Be fruitful and increase in number and fill the water in the seas, and let the birds increase on the earth." (Genesis 1: 20)

When God created the birds and fish, he put them in the natural environment designated for them. Now, when God came to create men let's look at the place where he put him. "And the Lord God formed the man from the dust of the ground and breathed into his nostrils the breath of life, and the man became a living being." (Genesis 2: 7)

Now the Lord had planted a garden in *Eden. What is Eden?* A place of pleasure, paradise, a place of glorious living, a place of delight or pleasure to the senses; a place where the temperature is right, the weather is good. The food is also delicious. A place where the temperature is right - have you ever wondered why when it is hot people complain, and when it is cold people complain? This is because when God first created man, he put him in a place where the temperature was perfect, a place of perfect living. Now we come to IVF and embryo freezing. A lot of people say the embryo does not have life yet. It doesn't feel pain so it is all right to freeze it. May I ask you a question? Are those embryos alive? Are they capable of becoming human beings? If you reply yes, it means they can feel pain as well.

I can boldly tell you that when you take a creature and place it in an environment contrary to its nature it is morally wrong. When you take a human embryo and freeze it for years, you are taking the laws of God into your own hands. The Bible says the secret things belong to God. The things that are revealed belong to us and our children. (Deuteronomy 29: 29) Even doctors will tell you that they know very little in these issues that concern fertility. The doctors clearly admit that freezing embryos and IVF have their setbacks as the children born as a result could in later years be deformed or have disabilities that are incurable. The Bible says God himself determines the time every human being is to be born and the exact place in which they should live. (Acts 17: 26)

When you freeze babies and want to bring them out at your own convenience, you are playing God. In freezing embryos you have now taken the place of God and you are creating life by yourselves. You have taken the secret things of God into your hands. I want you to know that, because something solves a problem or looks good, it does not mean that we, as children of God, should dabble in it.

In every situation, we must let the Holy Spirit guide and lead us in the wisdom of God. God designed a perfect environment for a child in the womb of its mother; any other system that takes that child out of that environment and places it in any other environment is in direct opposition to the laws of God.

This is what I will advise my fellow Christian brothers and sisters to do. If you have dabbled in this worldly practice, repentance is in order. You must go on your knees and ask God to forgive you and also ask God to take such a child to become His own and heal every hidden disorder or abnormality that may exist.

God is faithful and just, and He is merciful, and He will forgive you and bless that child. ***Do it today!*** While there is still time. God bless you. If you are not a Christian, God does not condemn you if you do these things; God wants you to come to Him and He Himself will bless you and guide you. God loves you. He will forgive you and help you if you ask Him in faith.

What of donor insemination and egg donation for the Christian couple?

What is donor insemination?

This is where sperm from a donor rather than the husband is placed into the woman's vagina or womb, with the intention of fertilising one of her eggs. Love-making is not involved but tubes are the means used to transfer the sperms.

This method is used when:

♦ The man is not producing enough sperm or not producing at all.
♦ Where the man is carrying a genetic disease that could be passed on to his children.
♦ Where women who are not married wish to have children.

What is egg donation?

Egg donation is usually embarked on when the woman is unable to produce her own eggs. These could be as a result of:

1. Her ovaries failing to work properly due to cancer treatment or some other problems.
2. Where the woman have no ovaries at all.
3. Where the man or woman cannot produce viable sperm or egg and a donated embryo is the only way for the woman to become pregnant.

To overcome these problems the woman now receives an egg from another woman, which could be used for fertilisation with her partner's sperms and the embryo placed in her womb.

What the Bible says

The first thing that we should get clear is that God created a man and woman to live together as one and multiply and have children in a happy environmental setting. A woman who does not want to marry should not be asking for sperm donation to enable her have children. Having children according to the way ordained by God is to be commenced after marriage. Where a husband and wife decide to employ the sperm or eggs of a stranger, who is not a party to their marriage, to father or be the mother to their children, this the Bible calls adultery. Why?

Is it adultery, even though physical intercourse is not involved? Where two strangers enter into an agreement to produce an illegitimate child, the act is illegal and immoral before God.

Reasons

The child born to such couples belong to another man or woman, not to the wife or husband.

No one knows what kind of blood is being introduced into the family

The Bible says the sins of the fathers are visited upon the children to the fourth generation. Whose child is your wife going to be carrying? It could be the child of a mass murderer or even a Satanist or a person with a deadly disease and such weakness could be brought into your home. I know that God loves us and wants to bless everyone but the children of God must act in wisdom.

A lot of precautions are taken to prevent the receptor knowing who the donor is. Yet it is possible the unknown donor could trace the family and this could lead to blackmail.

The child may find out the circumstances of their birth and this could lead to low self-image, rejection or rebellion in later years. The husband or wife may, after that child is born, feel resentful towards the child because they know the child is not of their own seed.

Many Christians are asking questions on this issue and want to know what the Bible says. But from the scriptures it is quite clear that this is a reckless act of man. The Bible warns us of "taking the laws of God into our hands". "Has not the Lord God made them one? In flesh and spirit they are his. And why one? Because he was seeking godly offspring. So guard yourself in your spirit and do not break faith with the wife of your youth." (Malachi 2: 15) God made them one in flesh and spirit because he desires godly offspring from the two. Will you call the seed of a stranger godly offspring. Is that the plan of God for man?

Donor insemination or egg donation is committing adultery in the spirit. A life is created when the sperm from the male meets with the eggs of the woman. God made this possible in a healthy marriage environment. Where this event is done outside a marital relationship, making it possible for a woman to bear another man's child other than her husband, this is adultery; it also gives a single woman an opportunity to have a child without a husband and this contradicts the commands of God. He who gave the command, gave it to a man and woman, and not to a single lady. Why are we encouraging single ladies to have children on their own without marriage? This is wrong before our God. Adultery is a sin involving the body. The Bible warns us to, "flee from sexual immorality, all other sins a man commits are outside his body, but he who sins sexually sins against his own body." (1 Corinthians 6: 18)

Donor insemination or egg donation is a sexual sin, in the sense that the sperm or eggs of a stranger are being introduced into the vagina of another man's wife. Our Lord Jesus Christ said: "But I tell you that anyone who looks at a woman lustfully has already committed adultery with her in his heart." (Matthew 5: 28) So if only looking amounts to adultery what will you call the exchange of sperm and egg? This is not an issue to be looked on lightly, but it is an issue where you must honestly seek the face of the Holy Spirit and the Word of God. For a husband and wife to sit down and agree that the wife be impregnated by another woman's egg or another man's seed is a deliberate act of adultery because it is coming from their heart (from the spirit). For a single woman to sit down and decide to bring a child into the world by receiving the sperm of a stranger is a reckless act likely to incur divine displeasure. The Bible warns us thus - "marriage should be honoured by all, and the marriage bed kept pure, for God will judge the adulterer and all the sexually immoral." (Hebrews 13: 4) Where you have gone wrong as a couple, repent and ask God to forgive you for your ignorance; God is merciful and forgives if we repent.

This is completely different from adoption where the couple have no part in the existence of that child. Let's look at adoption.

What of adoption?

Adoption or to adopt is to take by choice into a new relationship, to bring up voluntarily a child of other parents as one's own child). Many people today have adopted children without home, orphans to give them a loving home and a new family. Adoption is good and right as long as a Christian couple does not consider it as an alternative to having their own children. One couple wrote that God wanted them to adopt; that's why he did not bless them with their own biological children. This statement is wrong in itself. While it is good to adopt, to assume that God has denied you children because he wants you to adopt is wrong. If God does this it means His Word to us, "That sons are a heritage from the Lord, children a reward from him" (Psalms 127: 3) is wrong. God cannot promise us something and deny us that thing. That is not the nature and character of God. Whatever he says, h e stands by it, and he does not change His mind. When you adopt a child and bring that child into your home, the protection and glory of God overshadows that child because you have taken that child as your own child. Be sensitive to the Holy Spirit to direct you, concerning the prayer needed for such a child, because there could be family weakness that child may have inherited from their biological parents which could surface later in life, if not dealt with properly in prayers. God himself says he is the father of the orphans. If God is the father of orphans, it in effect makes these little ones our responsibility to make sure they are well cared for and loved. I have just written briefly on this issue to let the Christian couple know that adoption is a godly and right thing to do; yet, at the same time, to let the Christian couple also know that even if they adopt, the will of God for them in Christ does not change. He still desires to bless them with their own biological children if that's what they desire. Esther, one of the great women of God, who was used by God to deliver His people at a trying time was an adopted child. (Esther 2: 7)

I am not a Christian - what are my chances with God on this issue?

Many of you reading this book may not be Christians and may be wondering if God can help you and hear your prayers because you are not a Christian. Well today I want you to know that God loves you and cares about you. If you make a decision today to accept Jesus Christ in your life as your Lord and Saviour, as soon as you say those prayers written in this book on how to accept Jesus, you instantly become a child of God.

God now gives you the same right as me and those who have served him for all their years. You are able to confess Jesus as Lord and take your place in God's plan for your life. The promises of God concerning having children and healing automatically become yours. Let us look at a woman who was not a Christian but made a decision to serve God and what God did in her life.

Setting up a blessing after infertility - Ruth

This story will challenge and encourage you and let you know that God is faithful to His Word and that the curse can be reversed and a blessing set up.

Under the leadership of the Holy Spirit we now take a journey through the pages of the Bible to the Book of Ruth to meet two great women and also to have a chat with Ruth, who rejected the curse of her people and set herself up for a blessing. Before we chat with Ruth I personally want to tell Naomi that she is a great woman of God. She lived a life worthy of emulation by all children of God. I can boldly write that without a Naomi there could never have been a Ruth. Naomi lived a godly life. She lived the life our Lord Jesus asked us to live; let your light shine before men, that they shall see it and give glory to our Father in Heaven.

Naomi was that light, her strength, quietness, and faithfulness to God produced faith in the heart of Ruth, which moved Ruth to accept God in her life. Now we see Ruth; she was a Moabite woman, who married Naomi's son. After ten years of marriage her husband died. (Ruth 1: 4-5)

Naomi who was living in Moab, now decided to go back home to her people in Israel. She told Ruth to go back to her people since her husband was dead. Ruth found her heart closely tied to Naomi and she refused to be separated from her in the pathway that lay before her, choosing to share whatever the future might hold in store for the one on whom her love was set. The Moabites were cursed people, they were fleshy and carnal. We read in Numbers 22: 6, how the King of Moab sent for a prophet to come and curse God's people; the prophet could not curse them, but only bless them. When they could not entice this prophet to curse God's people, they then enticed God's people to fall into sexual sins. The Bible says, "while Israel was staying in Shittim, the men began to indulge in sexual immorality with Moabite women, who invited them to the sacrifice of their god, so Israel joined in worshipping the Baal of Poer and the anger of God burned against them." (Numbers 25: 1-3)

Ruth was coming from this type of background and when Naomi told her to go back to her people she now said these words to Naomi and set up a family blessing for herself and the whole world. "Where you go I will go; where you stay I will stay, your people will be my people and your God will be my God." (Ruth 1: 16)

Alleluia! What a woman! The light of God had shone into her spirit. She rejected all that was not of God and chose to serve God and be with God's people. All I can say to this, is that this type of harvest in the kingdom of God can never be obtained by the witness of the lips; our lives must be vindicated and reinforced by the witness of our lives. Some daughters-in-law do not have a loving relationship and are always in a hurry to leave the company of their mothers-in-law because of their behaviour, but Naomi was different. What she preached she lived. May this example be our testimony in Jesus' name.

Now we see the blessing that followed Ruth's statement: "So Boaz took Ruth and she became his wife; then he went to her and the Lord enabled her to conceive and give birth to a son." (Ruth 4: 13) The Holy Spirit told me Ruth was barren until she gave her heart to the Lord. She was under the curse of infertility for ten years of her marriage to Naomi's son. Note the words: - *"The Lord enabled her to conceive."* What does the word enable mean? It means to provide with the means or opportunity; to make possible, practical or easy. God made it easy for her. It was Ruth who had the fault; she was infertile but God healed her, and made it possible for her to conceive. The day she said these words, *"your God shall be my God"*, she set up an eternal blessing which the whole world including you and I are still enjoying. She gave birth to a son, Obed, who was the father of Jesse, who was the father of David, through whom Jesus Christ came into the world.

God used that family to accomplish His plan and purpose on the earth and because of her wisdom she reversed the curse on her life.

She had a whole book in the Bible named after her, so you see God is no respecter of persons. If you come to him He will bless you even more than you thought or imagined.

Chapter Seventeen

The Fatherhood Of God

What is a father?

The dictionary describes father as a male parent of a child. He is also the first person of the Trinity, God; a man who relates to another in a way suggesting the relationship of father and child, to beget, to give rise to, to initiate, to accept responsibility for. In this chapter, I would like to discuss with you the fatherhood of God. Many of us have never thought of God as our Father, but God is the one who created us in His image. In the book of Genesis it reads: "So God created man in His image. In the image of God He created him; male and female, He created them. (Genesis 1: 27) You and I are made in the image of God. God is our Heavenly father, when you look at yourself, what you see is the image of God. You are created in *His* image. Today I want to let you know that God loves you and wants you to know that he is your Father. Our Lord Jesus Christ himself, in speaking about the Fatherhood of God, shared one of the most powerful Bible accounts with us to let us understand the Fatherhood of God.

Through the leadership of the Holy Spirit, I will like us to look into the Bible to read about the Fatherhood of God and even as you read I pray that the Holy Spirit quicken your understanding to comprehend and understand the Father who loves you and is calling out for you to come home.

> There was a man who had two sons. The younger one said to his father, "Father, give me my share of the estate." So he divided his property between them. Not long after that, the

younger son got together all he had, set off for a distant country and there squandered his wealth on wild living. After he had spent everything, there was a severe famine in that whole country and he began to be in need, so he went and hired himself out to a citizen of that country, who sent him to his field to feed pigs. He longed to fill his stomach with the pods the pigs were eating, but no-one gave him anything.

When he came to his senses, he said, "How many of my father's hired men have food to spare, and here I am starving to death! I will set out and go back to my father and say to him: Father I have sinned against heaven and against you, I am no longer worthy to be called you son; make me like one of your hired men." So he got up and went to his father. But while he was still a long way off, his father saw him and was filled with compassion for him; he ran to his son, threw his arms around him and kissed him. The son said to him, "Father, I have sinned against heaven and against you. I am no longer worthy to be called your son." But the father said to his servants, "Quick! Bring the best robe and put it on him. Put a ring on his finger and sandals on his feet. Bring the fattened calf and kill it. Let's have a feast and celebrate. For this son of mine who was dead is alive again; he was lost and is found." So they began to celebrate. (Luke 15: 11-24)

Throughout the ministry of our Lord Jesus Christ, he was found among the needy, the sinners, prostitutes and those less privileged. The Pharisees and scribes murmured, saying, "This man received sinners and eats with them." He had already made a bad name for himself because of this. These Pharisees could not understand why Jesus received and talked with prostitutes and outcasts of any kind. It was a constant surprise to them that these people also loved Jesus. Those outcasts and needy people loved the Lord. In this parable of the lost son, Jesus explained why he loved these people. He told of the pain and love in the fatherhood of God. He told them of the father who had two sons and had lost one and because one was lost, he was more concerned about the lost son than the one who was safe at home. The point here is that something was temporarily lost, something of great value to the owner, and because it was lost, he was greatly concerned just as we would be if we lost a son.

For many of you reading this book, if you do not know Jesus Christ as your Lord and Saviour or God as your Father, I want to tell you plainly today, that you are the missing son or daughter that God is looking for. He is calling you to come back home to Him. He is the father who is sore for that lost child in a far away country. You may not care or have thought much about God and how He feels but I have now learnt that it is the one who loses the loved one that suffers most. It is the father or mother who suffers when their boy or girl has gone off into the world to pleasure him or herself. Oh, the pain and agony of a father or mother who would suffer any pain in this life, go to any length if it were possible, if by any means he or she could save that thankless child and bring him or her home! I want to relate this to you men and women who desire to have children today. What will you do if twenty years from now this same child you suffered to give birth to then turns his back on you and says: "No way, daddy/mummy; I don't love you any more." How will you feel? What will you do? Think about it. Will you give up on that son or daughter? Even if you will, God has not given up on you. The Bible says:

> "Can a mother forget the baby at her breast and have no compassion on the child she has borne? Though she may forget, I will not forget you! See, I have engraved you on the palms of my hands; your walls are ever before me." (Isaiah 49: 15-16)

He still wants you back, he is diligently searching for you until he finds you; he does not console himself for your loss by fellowship with people who have never sinned, he does not content himself by using others to fill in the blank. He is not a great employer of labour who can have fresh hands to take the place of the failures. No, says our Saviour Jesus, he is the Father, he wants you, he misses you. He goes after that which is lost until he finds it. The prodigal son came to his senses and decided to go back home to his father; he knew in his father's house he would have food to eat and shelter over his head. Today I also want to ask those of you who do not know him yet, will you come to your senses? Will you go back to the Father whose arms are empty, who aches for you, whose eyes are full of tears because of his love for you? Will you come home today?

The prodigal son thought that when he went back home his father would treat him like one of his hired men, but how wrong he was. As soon as the father saw him coming, the father ran to him and said to his servants, "Quick, bring the best robe and put it on him, put a ring on his finger and sandals on him. Bring the fattened calf and kill it. Let's have a feast and celebrate, for this son of mine was dead but is now alive again; he was lost but now is found." So they began to celebrate. (Luke 15: 22-24) I have spoken to many people on the road as I go along, telling them about Jesus Christ and the love of God and they comment with statements like: "Oh, there are too many people in the world, why would God care about me? But I want you to know He cares. His arms are waiting for you to come home to Him. When the prodigal son came home he found all he was looking for at home; there was food to keep him warm, sandals for his feet, clothes on his back and a welcome party, and love too. When you come home, you will be coming back to the family of God, the God who said, *"In my house there shall be none barren."* (Deuteronomy 7: 14); the God who said, "there shall be no sickness in my house for I am the Lord who sent my word and it heals you." (Psalms 107: 20); the God who said, "I will create the fruit of your lips." (Isaiah 57: 19) That is the house you are coming back to. Our Lord Jesus Christ spoke these words about the Father's love. "Fear not little children, it is your Father God's pleasure to give you the kingdom.

All these words are most comforting to the children, if they believe them. But what of the Father - he wants *you* back. I have written powerful books on infertility and creative miracles - these books are written by the Holy Spirit himself to bring you healing and restoration and blessing beyond measure.

But going beyond all these blessings, listen to the revelation of the Father's heart not told by me or any man not even by the apostles, but by the only begotten of God, Jesus Christ who is in the bosom of the Father. He has revealed that it is God's loss more than yours when you go astray, that God suffers more than you suffer by your godless life, that he cares more than you care for your return to good. This may shock you but it is the truth; it may sound incredible to you and yet it ought not to be if we look, as our Lord Jesus bids us do, at the reflectionoof God in all human love.

Today I advise you to come back home - the Father's arms are open, waiting for you. Come back home. You may say, how do I come back home? Read on to the next chapter - **Who Is Jesus Christ?** and find out how.

Chapter Eighteen

Who Is Jesus Christ?

The love of God led him to give Jesus Christ for the sake of you and me. His searching for us made him send Jesus to die on the Cross for you and for me. The Bible says that, "God so loved the world that He gave His only begotten son, that whoever believes in Him shall not perish but have eternal life. For God did not send His son into the world to condemn it but to save the word through Him." (John 3: 16-17) Jesus came into the world to redeem us from the power of sin and death.

The will to choose abused

God created Adam from the dust of the ground and he became a living being. Now God planted a garden in the east, in Eden and there he put the man he had formed and the Lord God made all kinds of trees grow out of the ground - trees that were pleasing to the eye and good for food. In the middle of the garden were the tree of life and the tree of the knowledge of good and evil. The Lord God took the man and put him in the garden of Eden to work it and take care of it. And the Lord commanded the man, "You are free to eat from any tree in the garden, but you must not eat from the tree of the knowledge of good and evil, for when you eat of it you will surely die." (Genesis 2: 7-9, 15-17)

God created Adam with a unique ability to choose. He gave him free will and told Adam specifically, "You are free to eat from any tree in the garden but you must not eat from the tree of knowledge of good and evil, for the day you eat of it you will surely die." (Genesis 2: 17)

What kind of death was God talking about?

This was not physical death but spiritual death. Yet Adam did not obey God, for the Bible records that "Adam and his wife ate of these fruit that God had commanded them not to eat. When the woman saw that the fruit of the tree was good for food and pleasing to the eye and also desirable for gaining wisdom, she took some and ate of it. She also give some to her husband, who was with her and he ate of it." (Genesis 3: 6) That disobedience brought death to the whole of mankind - why? - because we all were in Adam when he disobeyed God's instruction. You say: "How can that be possible?" Medically, it is a fact that a man produces ten million sperm cells a day in his testicles and each of these sperm is genetically unique. So in just six months only one man produces enough sperm to populate the whole world.

There is no doubt from the Bible account, that it is, "from one man that God made every nation of men, that they should inhabit the whole earth and He determined the times set for them and the exact place where they should live." (Acts 17: 26) There are a lot of theories about the origin of man but the Bible does not speculate on this issue. It is clear and simply written down for those who desire to know the truth.

After Adam's fall, we all fell with him because we all were in him. There was no other way for mankind to be saved again because the law requires that everything be cleansed with blood because without the shedding of blood, there is no forgiveness. (Hebrews 9: 22) Jesus came into the world, led a sinless life in the world, and he shed His sinless blood on the Cross as an offering to redeem us from the sin committed by Adam. The Bible says

> Therefore, just as sin entered the world through one man, and death through sin, and in this way death came to all men, because all sinned - for before the law was given, sin was in the world. But sin is not taken into account when there is no law. Nevertheless death reigned from the time of Adam to the time of Moses, even over those who did not sin by breaking a command, as did Adam, who was a pattern of the one to come. But the gift is not like the trespass, for if many died by the trespass of the one man, how much more did God's grace and the gift that came by the one man, Jesus Christ, overflow to the many! (Romans 5: 12-16)

Adam brought sin into the world, Jesus brought the Grace of God into the world. Jesus came into the world, died on the Cross, shed His sinless blood on the Cross to redeem you and me from the sin committed by Adam. In His death he paid the price for the sin of all mankind; the curtain of sin that separated us from God was removed forever; Christ took our place and paid the price for you and me. Jesus Christ was sent by God. Mankind had fallen into sin and rebellion. Mankind had turned his back on God. "We all like sheep, have gone astray. Each of us has turned to his own way." (Isaiah 53: 6) No man sought God any more, sin had separated us from God. God had to do something to restore the fellowship between him and man. This made him send Jesus to come down to the earth and die on the Cross to redeem us from sin and death. Before we look at what Jesus did for us, let's look at the old covenant.

Old covenant priest

In the old covenant the high priest was the mediator before God and the people. He was the one who offered the animal sacrifice day after day first for his own sins and then for the sins of the people. He carried the blood of animals into the most Holy Place as a sin offering and the bodies of the animals were burnt outside the camp. This he did day in day out, yet the blood of goat and bull could not take away sins, they remained an annual reminder of sin.

The high priest of Jesus Christ

When Jesus came as a high priest of good things that are already here, he went through the greater and more perfect tabernacle that is not man-made, that is to say, not created by man. He did not enter by means of the blood of goats and calves; but he entered the most Holy place once and for all by His own blood, having obtained eternal redemption. The blood of goats and bulls and the ashes of a heifer sprinkled on those who were ceremonially unclean sanctified them so that they were outwardly clean.

> How much more, then will the blood of Christ, who through the eternal Spirit, offered himself unblemished to God, cleanse our consciences from acts that lead to death, so that we may serve the Living God? (Hebrews 9: 11-14)

When Jesus came into the world, he saw that the sacrifice of animals for sin offering could not save mankind, so he decided to offer His own sinless body on the Cross and shed His blood to cleanse us forever from sin. This he did by dying on the Cross for us. Before Jesus could die on the Cross he had to live for thirty-three years on earth, and yet

He was still without sin. The life of our Lord Jesus in its final perfection was a perpetual message to men concerning their unfitness to enter the divine presence. He lived a life of unbroken fellowship with God, which we know we cannot do. His fellowship resulted from His being well pleasing to God. (Luke 3: 22) His life on earth was acceptable to God, He did not fail or disappoint God so he was qualified to become the Saviour of all mankind. Nothing has ever separated man and God except sin. Jesus was sinless and so lived with God, but His death on the Cross dealt with our sin and made it possible for us to return to God. Our access to God at all times and under all circumstances is open.

Draw near to Christ

Christ can only complete His work of saving men when they draw near to God through him. For Christ to do this there are two things which has priesthood is based upon. First we must make ourselves available to His priesthood and secondly submit ourselves to His authority. And in doing this we will find complete salvation for all things in him. It is only when men draw near that the priesthood of Jesus is operative in all their continuous activities.

Intercession

One of His duties as the Bible records is intercession, continuous praying without ceasing, because Christ is praying for us. Our drawing near to him keeps us within the cover of His prayer, and through this intercession, we are being perfected and strengthened from day to day. As this nearness is maintained, Christ our great high priest is the mediator through whom all the resources of the divine wisdom, strength and grace of God are communicated to us. We are being strengthened in our inner selves, growing up into Him; in all things our salvation to the uttermost is complete, to depart from nearness to God separates us from the protection of our high priest. This is a truth we must never forget. Standing alone, we are liable to be discouraged. But that brings us to the second truth, and that is that our nearness to God is through Him. It is through Him we draw near, and it is through Him that we abide in nearness. Thus the two places of His priesthood are in view. The first is atoning, by which we draw near and abide in nearness. The second is intercessory and perfecting, that operates as we are near to God through His atoning work.

Let us draw near

"Let us draw near." (Hebrews 10: 22) Today I want to encourage you to draw near to Jesus Christ. Why? - because he has created the access which we need to get into the presence of God. This possibility of approach and access is the supreme fact resulting from the work of our great high priest. The one thing we are called to do is to draw near. There is no reason why we should not do so.

Every sin dealt with

Everything which excluded men from God was put away by Christ at His death on the Cross. The Bible records that on the day Christ was crucified, the sun stopped shining and the curtain of the temple was torn in two. (Luke 23: 45) Why was this curtain torn into two? This curtain was a symbol of that which had excluded man from God, through sin. In its rent condition it was the symbol of the open way to God.

Come the way you are

Therefore the appeal to us is not a call to prepare ourselves, or to make a way for ourselves to God, it simply says come, draw near, enter in. This invitation to come in is through our great high priest; this we can all do by going in faith, without fear. Our Lord Jesus Christ in John 6: 35 declared:

> "I am the bread of life. He who comes to me will never go hungry, and he who believes in me will never be thirsty. All that the Father gives me will come to me and whoever comes to me I will never drive away. For I have come down from Heaven not to do my will but to do the will of Him who sent me. And this is the will of Him who sent me, that I shall lose none of all that He has given me, but raise them up at the last day. For my Father's will is that everyone who looks to the son and believes shall have eternal life, and I will raise him up at the last day." (John 6: 35-40)

God's will was why Jesus came to the earth to give both physical and spiritual life to those who believe. He also promises that he will never reject anyone who comes to him. Many people think they need to stop sinning, go take a holy bath or do something before they can come to Jesus. Today I want to tell you, you don't need to do anything to come to him. Nothing is good enough except for you to accept His love and grace which he freely offers to those who believe in him. Most of the blessings written down in these books belong to those who belong to Christ because, you see, it is He who paid the price to redeem us from the curses of the law which were hanging over us. On His death and resurrection on the third day, Jesus destroyed for ever all curses and sin that hung over all humans. But to avail yourself of this finished work you must come to Him and accept what He has done for you.

Salvation

To accept him as your Lord and Saviour the Bible says that the Word is near you: It is in your mouth and in your heart; that is the word of faith we are proclaiming that if you confess with your mouth "Jesus is Lord", and believe in your heart that God raised him from the dead you will be saved. For it is with your heart that you believe and are justified, and it is with your mouth that you confess and are saved. When you confess Jesus as Lord and Saviour you can pray in your own way, any way you know how, the simpler the better; the most important thing is your heart's condition.

Confession

Father, I come to you in the name of Jesus. I confess that I have sinned against you and lived in sin. Father, I repent of my sins and by your power I will no longer be a servant of sin. Father, make me your child. I believe that Jesus died on the Cross and that he shed His blood for me and that he rose from the dead on the third day. I confess and accept the Lord Jesus as my Lord and Saviour Lord; come into my life. Give me new hope and power to live for you. Wash me with your blood and sanctify me with your word and fill me with your Holy Spirit, to your praise and glory. Father, I thank you for making me your child. In the name of Jesus Christ of Nazareth, Amen!

Right standing with God

Immediately after the confession you now have right standing with God. The Bible says once we are justified through faith, we have peace with God through our Lord Jesus Christ, through whom we have gained access by faith into this grace in which we now stand. And we rejoice in the hope of the glory of God. Accepting Jesus as Lord, the Bible says, "as many as receive him, to them he gave the power to become the sons of God, even to them that believe in His name. (John 1: 12) Once you have accepted Jesus Christ you now have a right standing with God and you are now born of the Spirit. This is the new birth, it gives you right standing with God.

He gives you the same benefits as those saved many years ago

Once you have accepted Jesus Christ as your Lord and Saviour all the benefits of the kingdom of God become available to you at the same moment; nowhere else can you receive such privileges. If a company employs you today, there is no way they will pay you the same amount or give you the same benefit as those who have worked forty or fifty years with them. But glory to God Almighty, He is no respecter of persons, the blood of Jesus qualifies you immediately for all of God's benefit.

Matthew 20

Our Lord Jesus Christ himself explained this himself in Matthew 20.

> For the kingdom of Heaven is like a landowner who went out early in the morning to hire men to work in His vineyard. He agreed to pay them a denarius for the day and sent them into His vineyard. About the third hour he went out and saw others standing in the market place doing nothing. He told them "You also go and work in my vineyard, and I will pay you whatever is right." So they went. He went again at about the sixth hour and the ninth hour and did the same.

> About the eleventh hour he went out and found still others standing around. He asked them, "Why have you been standing here all day doing nothing? "Because no one has hired us," they answered. He said to them, "You also go and work in my vineyard." When the evening came, the owner of the vineyard said to his foreman, "Call the workers and pay them their wages, beginning with the last ones hired and going to the first. The workers who were hired about the eleventh hour came and each received a denarius. So when those who were hired first came, they expected to receive

more but each one of them also received a denarius. When they received it, they began to grumble against the land owner. "Those men who were hired last worked only one hour," they said, "and you have made them equal to us who have borne the burden of the work and the heat of the day." But he answered one of them "Friends I am not being unfair to you. Didn't you agree to work for a denarius? Take your pay and go. I want to give the man who was hired last the same as I gave you. Don't I have the right to do what I want with my own money? Or are you envious because I am generous? So the last will be the first, and the first will be the last." (Matthew 20: 1-16)

Reading through this Bible account spoken by our Lord Jesus Christ himself, I want to encourage you to come to God, for you have right standing with him now; what he will give to those who have walked with him a hundred years he also gives to you. Many people may not like this; as you see, the labourers who came first were not happy when the land owner paid all the workers the same amount. They wanted more; a lot of people may tell you, "Oh, you are a new Christian, you must do this and that." I will advise you to come to God yourself. He will fill you with His Holy Spirit who will direct you and guide you in all your ways. He will help you when you need help. He himself will direct you to a good church where you will grow in His Word and have a family in the body of Christ. He himself will place the right people in your life, who will not try to intimidate you but will help you to walk in the way of the truth to seek God for yourself.

A new baby

God's desire is for you to grow up in His grace and come closer to him. Take an example; when your baby is born, you will nurse that baby for about one year or more. When it starts to walk, you will encourage your baby to take steps towards mummy or daddy. You are happy when he or she does. So God also is happy each time you take a step towards Him. Your steps may not be firm yet but He is happy just seeing you take those steps. When the baby starts talking you are happy to see the baby talk; you encourage the baby to talk to you. Even though the words may not make sense to others it's amazing how parents, especially mothers, always understand what their babies are saying. So God wants to hear you yourself speaking to him, even though you may think you are not good enough or don't know what to say. God himself, like the mother, understands the baby. God also understands you. Even when you don't say a word, he is the "God who searches the heart and mind." (Psalm 7: 9) He knows what is in your heart.

The man born blind (John 9: 1-38)

A wise decision was made by the man born blind, whose Bible accounts I used in male congenital disorders, in this book. Jesus went along the road one day and he saw a man born blind; he went to him, made some mud with his saliva and put it on the man's eyes and said to him, "Go, wash in the pool of Siloma." So the man went and washed and came back able to see. When the man went home, his neighbours and those who used to see him sit and beg asked, "Isn't this the same man who use to sit and beg?" Some claimed he was. Others said, "No, he only looks like him, but he himself insisted, "I am the man." "How then were your eyes opened?" they demanded. He replied, "The man called Jesus made some mud and put it on my eyes. He told me to go and wash and then I could see." "Where is this man?" they asked him. "I don't know" he said.

Watch out for the negative critics

There are people who will pick up this book and criticise and try to analyse with their brains what has been written. These people are those who have never prayed for anyone in their lifetime. They are those who have never sought God's face to make them a blessing to others in their generation. These people have never done anything to bless anyone in their life; all they do is criticise what others have done to bless their generation. Don't listen to them; this man was healed immediately.

The Pharisees investigate the healing (John 9: 13-41)

This man was brought to the Pharisees; the day on which Jesus healed the man was the Sabbath. They questioned the man as to how he had received his sight. The man told them what Jesus did. Some of the Pharisees said, "This man is not from God, for he does not keep the Sabbath. Here we see a man born blind receiving his sight, yet all the religious leaders could think about was keeping the Sabbath laws. They were not bothered that a whole man had been restored to full health; they did not care that a man who had become a miserable sight in his locality was now well - all they cared about was Sabbath laws. For you, my readers, if you really have a need that only God can meet, please don't listen to those who do not really care about you. When you come to such people, they will criticise the Word that God has graciously sent to bless you, and they will discourage you and let you go empty. Immediately you leave they will forget you ever came, so be careful what and who you listen to. No negative critic ever cares about the benefits of others. All they do is pick up another man's work and destroy it like this Pharisee in our Lord's day on earth. They continued to argue with this man as to how he got his sight through healing; when they saw they were losing the argument they became angry and sent for the man's parents.

The Pharisees and the man's parents

The Jews still did not believe that he had been blind and had received his sight until they sent for the man's parents. "Is this your son?" they asked. "Is this the one you said was born blind? How is it that now he can see?" "We know he is our son," the parents answered, "and we know that he was born blind, but how he can see now, or who opened his eye, we do not know. Ask him; he is of age, he can answer for himself." His parents said this because they were afraid of the Jews, for they had already decided that anyone who acknowledged that Jesus was the Christ would be put out of the synagogue. That was why his parents said, "He is of age; ask him." (John 9: 18-23) The Pharisees thought they could intimidate the parents through fear either to deny their son's identity or the fact that he was born blind, but they did neither. How could they? Almost everyone knew this blind man and the plight of his family. They admitted that this man was their son and they also knew with sorrow that he had been born blind, but beyond that they proceeded with anxiety. They declined to give further evidence; ignorance of the miracle was pleaded. What a pity that these parents, at a time of great criticism, refused to stand by the testimony of their son. These parents were people of compromise. Instead of bearing their testimony to the honour of the One who had delivered their son from blindness, they squirmed and dodged, in order to curry favour with the Pharisees, they "passed the load" to their son and slid out of all responsibility in the matter. Jesus had said, "This man's blindness was not due to his parents' sin," but their sin was to leave their son in the grip of blind religious leaders who had no sympathy whatever with the healer. Jesus said. "If you declare me before men, I will declare you before my father and the angels." (Matthew 25: 31) Time and time again I have seen this scripture work in my life. When circumstances look difficult, I have stood and declared God and his might and his ability to come through for me to the shame of those who opposed me or God's Word. This blind man's parents failed to declare God's works when they were supposed to.

The plea and boldness of the beggar

A second time they summoned the man who had been blind. "Give glory to God," they said. "We know that this man is a sinner." He replied, "Whether he is a sinner or not I don't know. One thing I do know. *I was blind and now I see!*" Then they asked him, "What did he do to you? How did he open your eyes?" He answered them, "I have told you already and you did not listen. Why do you want to hear it again?" Do you want to become his disciple too?" (John 9: 24-27) After the weakness and fear exhibited by the blind man's parents we must confront the bold act of this man that was blind but could now see. The Pharisees tried to intimidate him and entangle him in a religious controversy; the man however stuck to his straightforward story about his cure from blindness.

He stands true to Christ

He remained true to Christ in the face of persecution and opposition. He bore his faithful witness in the face of all threats from the religious leaders.

His testimony

Whether he is a sinner or not I do not know. One thing I do know is that "I was blind but now I see!" The man answered them thus; now that is remarkable - he didn't know where He came from, yet He opened his eyes. We know God does not listen to sinners. He listens to the godly man who does His will. Nobody has ever heard of opening the eyes of a man born blind. If this man were not from God, he could do nothing.

This man stood strong by his testimony; it is marvellous for its truth and straightforwardness. "I once was blind but now I see." He stood up boldly to the Pharisees and to their wilful opposition to what Christ had done for him. He could not understand why the miracle had not convinced them of the glory of His personality.

Judge right

This man did not yet know who Jesus was; but this man born blind, who had never read a single letter in his life, was able to judge more rightly than these religious leaders; these learned men who claimed to know everything could not discern the matters of the divine and the really spiritual things were beyond them. A bunch of so called learned men had spent a whole day arguing about the healing of a man who was born blind, condemning it and calling the healer a sinner. Here may I add that a spiritual layman may learn more of God in half an hour through the Holy Spirit than religious leaders. who do not have the Holy Spirit, can learn in a thousand years through their human wisdom and fleshy deliberations.

The unjust action of the Pharisees

As the man continued to talk to them they became angry and they replied him like this: "You were seeped in sin at birth, how dare you lecture us!" and they threw him out. They threw him out of their synagogue, forbidding him from worshipping there.

The man finds true worship

Jesus heard that they had thrown him out, and when he found him, he said, "Do you believe in the son of man?" "Who is he, sir?" the man asked, "Tell me so that I may believe in him. Jesus said, "You have now seen him; in fact he is speaking with you." While the blind religious leaders were dragging this man all over the place, the blind man's conception of Christ had been growing steadily. At first he did not know who he was; he only knew him as "the man they called Jesus"; later he knew him as a "Prophet" and then he moves on to know him as Jesus, "from God". While the Pharisees were steeped in their unbelief, this man goes on from one vision of the Saviour to another and grasps the truth of who Jesus is.

The eyes of his heart opens

This man on this very day received double sight - both physical and spiritual sight. As he saw the light of day, the light of the gospel of Jesus Christ also shone into his spirit. This man finally met Jesus when the Pharisees threw him out and Jesus asked him:

Our Lord's question

"Do you believe in the son of man?" This is the master's demand for faith. Such is always his demand. It is a personal demand, an intelligent demand, an absolutely necessary demand. This is one demand he makes on all men who come to him. This same demand he made on me and the same he will make of you. Do you believe in the son of man? Faith in Christ, "the sent of God", is an obligatory demand in the gospel. There can be no wavering in our conception of him. He is who he says he is, he who is "sent of the Father" to cure all blindness must be the centre of our faith.

The man's question

"Who is he sir?" the man asked; "tell me so that I may believe in him. (John 9: 36) The events of the past few hours have made the man ready to believe, with a heart full of gratitude and honesty he enquired as to who the Messiah is. He knew Jesus was from God, that testimony had already been given. Who then would know better than Jesus as to the origin and present dwelling of the Messiah. "Who is he, Lord? Where is the Lord? I want to believe, I am ready to receive. Having met you, I am anxious now to meet him from whom all blessings flow." It is not a question he desires merely to consider; his heart is now ready to go out in praise and worship to him who sends such marvellous servants to work such wonderful cures as he has experienced. His question is just and his soul yearns for satisfaction and rest in him. He has already had one taste of divine blessing, and his heart hungers for more and more.

Our Lord's revelation

"You have now seen him, in fact he is speaking with you." The man longed to meet the author of all blessings. He was nearer than he dreamed. Only a thin veil separated them, and soon even that would be thrown aside. "I am," Jesus said to him. The man's eyes were opened in order that he might see the Messiah, in order that he might know the Light of the world. "He is the one speaking with you." This is even better; he was not only seeing, but knowing the glory of the healer and his ears tingled with the sounds of heavenly music as the divine one talked.

The man's confession

Then the man said, "Lord, I believe and he worshipped him. (John 9: 38) His confession was short and simple. It was clear and decisive, it was full and it was life-giving. Here the argument and discouragement of that day from the religious leaders of being thrown out of the temple was over. The man:

Worshipped Christ

The man worshipped him and Christ accepted his worship. Only God must be worshipped. Accepting the man's worship, Jesus again acknowledged that He is God. The man adores, believes and is filled with joy. Not only has light flooded his blinded eyes, but light has burst upon his soul also.

It is one thing and a great thing to bring sight to blinded eyeballs; it is a better thing to bring eternal life to a darkened soul. "Once I was blind, now I see," the man declares.

True faith

True faith will always worship and follow the one who is worthy of worship. This was the act of overwhelming gratitude and reverence, an act that involved the exercise of great faith. So we see the religious leaders cast him out of their organised religion, straight into the open arms of Christ, the one who came for such a person as him. Today, I speak to you, my readers; if you have never known Jesus Christ for yourself, learn from this blind beggar whom Jesus gave light and sight to. This man at first did not know who Christ was but when he finally did, he bowed down and worshipped him. He became a believer. In this Bible account we see a man who was in an impossible situation, and needed help which no human being could provide for him, which no money could buy. Christ did it for him and he believed. I would encourage you to choose to go with Christ today. Christ gave this man help and he believed.

I will encourage you to accept Christ in your life today like this man did. The rewards are eternal.

Be encouraged

Throughout the Bible we find examples of God answering the prayers of desperate couples who were unable to have children. As my pastor would say: "Each time God opens the womb of a barren woman a miracle child comes out." Sarah and Abraham were barren for a 100 years and then Isaac came along, a child who was to be a blessing to God's people throughout the earth. Isaac and Rabekah had the same problem and later God blessed them with children. Jacob and Rachel waited for many years to have Joseph, but Joseph later became a prime minister and Deliverer for his people. Ruth the Moabite was barren for ten years but when she gave her life to God, God blessed her with a son named Obed through whom the Christ came into the world. So be encouraged you too carry seeds of destiny in you.

My prayer for you

Father, in the name of Jesus Christ, and the authority which you have given me, I stand in unison with my brother who is reading this book so that you will bless-him and grant him the desires of his heart that his joy may be complete. Father, I thank you that you remain the God of families and you love your people so much. Bring back joy and glory into the home of my brother, that all men will see that you alone are God. I bless you for his life and his family and I thank you that you have done it for him in the name of your son Jesus Christ. Amen. God bless you.

Chapter Ninteen

Prayer Points

- Stand upon Gods word that you are a joyous father of many children.
- Declare your victory over all manner of sperm count problems in Jesus name.
- Thank the Lord by faith that your sperm count is accurate.
- Declare your freedom from congenital disorders and hidden sickness and disease in your body.
- Praise the name of the Lord because you know he has made you a father of many children as promised in his word.
- Thank the Lord for turning all the negative reports you have received into positive. Condemn every tongue that has risen against you in accordance with Isaiah 54: 17.
- Declare in the name of Jesus that you are free from spiritual wickdness.
- Thank the Lord by faith that he has given you the desires of your heart.
- Thank the Lord for cleansing all your system of any effect of drug or alcohol abuse.
- Thank the Lord for renewing your strength and your splendour like those who are His own.
- Pray against the wickedness that destroys in the noonday light.
- Curse the root of every demonic entrance of the curse into your family.
- Receive a creative miracle by faith where it may be needed in your body.
- Declare in the name of Jesus that the Holy Spirit lives in you and bind any attempt of impotence to come near your body ever again.

Chapter Twenty

General daily Confession

I will extol the Lord at all times, his praise will always be on me lips. I bless you Father; I worship you Lord because you are the One who gives autumn and spring rains in season. My soul boasts in you Lord; let the afflicted hear and rejoice. Glorify the Lord with me; let us exalt his name together. I sought the Lord and he answered me, he delivered me from all my fears. I will continue to look up to the Lord and my face will remain radiant, my face can never be covered with shame (Psalms 34:1-4).

Your love for me O, Lord, riches to the heavens, your faithfulness to the skies. Your righteousness is like the mighty mountains, your justice like the great deep. O, Lord you preserve both man and beast. How priceless is your unfailingly love! Both high and low among men find refuge in the shadows of your wings. I feast in the abundance of your house; you give me drink from your river of delight. For with you is the fountain of life in your light I see light. Continue your love to those who know you, your righteousness to the upright in heart. (Psalm 36: 5-10). Because I delight myself in the Lord, he has given me the desires of my heart. (Psalm 37: 4). I am my Father's son; I belong to him. In his word he has promised that "there shall not be any male barren in his house." Christ has chosen me and ordained me that I should go and bring forth fruit, and that my fruit should remain, that whatever I ask the Father in His name, He will give it to me. (John 15:4-16). Today I part ways with infertility and declare that with the help of God I rise above infertility; I can boldly say, " I can do all things through Christ who strengthens me." (Philippians 4: 13). I am the father of many children.

My Father has given me the splendour of those who are His, and delivered from the curse of the law. Infertility is far from me. I am free from every genetic and generation problems.

I receive my healing from any hidden sickness or disease. I am the temple of God and the Holy Spirit lives in me. Any attempt of infertility in any form or disguise to come near my body ever again is bound. The power of God's Word has destroyed infertility forever because my body is sacred to God. (1st Corinthians 3: 16). I declare that by the stripes of Jesus Christ I am made whole. My sperm count its accurate, my penis is strong, erectile dysfunction is far from me. No growths or hidden infectious disease comes near me. The Lord is my refuge and my strength, an ever-present help in trouble. Therefore I will not fear, though the earth gives way and the mountains fall into the heart of the sea, for the Lord my God is the refuge and the strength of my life. (Psalm 46:1-2).

The Lord my God is robbed in majesty and is armed with strength, because I'm His son and precious to Him he has clothed my penis with His majesty and armed my penis with His strength. (Psalm 93: 1). I thank you Father for making me the father of many children in the name of Jesus. I plead the blood of Jesus Christ over every muscle and fibre of my being. I thank you Father for establishing your Word in my life. My home is full of the joy and the laughter of young children to your glory. I am singing and dancing because my Lord has turned me waste places into fertile grounds. (Isaiah 52: 9). The Lord has comforted me and redeemed my life from infertility. The Lord hath made bare his holy arm in the eyes of all the nations, and all the ends of the earth shall see the salvation of the Lord. (Isaiah 52: 9-10).

I have seen you in the sanctuary and beheld your power and your glory. Because your love is better than life, my lips will glorify you, I will praise you as long as I live and in your name I will lift up my hands. My soul will be satisfied as with the richest and most beautiful children, with singing lips my mouth we praise you. (Psalm 63:2-5). I thank you Father in Jesus name, amen.

Overcoming Infertility Collection
By Veronica Anusionwu

■   *Choosing Your Baby's Sex (Price: £2.95)*
Choosing Your Baby's Sex comes as a complement to Veronica Anusionwu's other two titles, "Man, You Are Not Infertile" and "Woman, You Are Not Infertile". In this book the author shares, from the very heart of God, all the information you need to choose the sex of your baby in order to make your joy complete, In this rich and fulfilling book, she also shares her own testimony of how she chose the sex of her own baby.

■   *Woman, You Are Not Infertile (Price: £10.99)*
The problem of infertility is a serious one, affecting over 100 million couples worldwide, yet at the very heart of God is an overwhelming desire to bless every woman with children. In this book Veronica Anusionwu wants us to turn away from the inadequate areas of medical research to the banquet of rich food prepared for us by Almighty God. All you have to do is say "Yes, God, I want to partake." This is a book written out of love, the kind of love that the Father has for his daughter when he would say, "Woman, you are not infertile, no matter what you have been through or what you have been told, I still want to bless you with children." Designed to assist women who are infertile, this book will also be useful to readers who wish to know more about God.

■   *Blissful Pregnancy, Pain Free Childbirth*
In this powerful book I am going to be sharing with you powerful revelations and Biblical knowledge; how you can have a problem-free pregnancy, having the most wonderful time of your life and bringing forth your baby without long hours of labour pain and painful contractions. This is childbirth the Holy Ghost way. I wish I had enjoyed such revelation knowledge when I had my own children. Register today at the Holy Ghost hospital for a wonderful and blessed nine months of blissful pregnancy and pain free labour.

■   *Oh! God Why All The Miscarriages?*
Veronica Anusionwu examines the issue of miscarriage, premature birth, still birth, incompetent cervix, birth defects from the spiritual perspective. She brings in the medical background of miscarriage before leading us into the Word of God for the solution. She answers questions on miscarriages and still birth, such as: Does God care when you lose a baby? Is it the will of God for us to suffer the loss of unborn babies? Is it the will of God for mankind, that a child be born with birth defects? In this book she brings the solution from the Word of God to help you keep that which God has freely given to you.

THE LORD'S WORD ON HEALING SERIES
Overcoming Infertility Collection
By Veronica Anusionwu
ORDER FORM

Yes, I want:

_____ copy/copies: "Man, You Are Not Infertile" @ £10.00 each

_____ copy/copies: "Woman, You Are Not Infertile" @ £10.99 each

_____ copy/copies: "Choosing Your Baby's Sex" @ £2.95 each

_____ copy/copies: "Oh God, Why All The Miscarriages?" @ £5.00

_____ copy/copies: "Who Said You Are Too Old To Conceive?" @ £4.99

_____ copy/copies: "Blissful Pregnancy, Pain Free Childbirth" @ £6.00

Please add £1.75 postage and packing per book. Cheques or postal orders should be made payable to: The Lords Word On Healing Publications.

Amount enclosed: _____

Name: _____

Address: _____

_____

_____

TESTIMONY FORM

The Bible says: "they overcome him by the blood of the lamb and by the word of their testimony." Your testimony is important to God and to man. Your testimony glorifies God. Your testimony gives hope to others facing the same situation - to know that if God did it for you He will do it for them. I will be doing a special testimony book in the near future. Make sure you send back your testimony to be included in this book. God bless you. You can photocopy this form and write your testimony and send it back to us or you can use a plain sheet of paper.

....
....
....
....
....
....
....
....
....
....
....
....
....
....
....
....
....
....
....
....
....

Mail to:

VERONICA ANUSIONWU, THE LORD'S WORD ON HEALING MINISTRIES PO BOX 24604, LONDON E2 9XA

Please kindly write to me to let me know how this book has helped you, I will be glad to hear from you. Veronica will be running faith clinics in the near future. To find out more about this clinic, please write, enclosing a self-addressed envelope. You can photocopy this form and fill it out and retun it to us.

THE LORD'S WORD ON HEALING MINISTRY

FAITH CLINIC APPLICATION FORM

The purpose of the faith clinic is to help those who may need someone to stand with them in prayer and faith to receive all they need from God. The faith clinic is designed to help build faith in God and Jesus Christ for those who need it.

Answer these questions truthfully. This will help us to determine what faith class you will need to attend.

DATE: _____

NAME: _____

AGE: _____

ADDRESS: _____
_____
_____

1) How long have you been trying for a baby?
_____

2) Have you undergone any medical check-up to diagonise the cause of infertility?

3) What was the diagnosis?

_____
_____
_____

4) Will you be willing to participate in a series of faith teachings from the Bible to build your faith to overcome your limitations? **Tick Box**
YES ☐   **NO** ☐

5) If you have been trying to conceive but have not gone through any medical check up.
YES ☐   **NO** ☐

6) Do you have any children?
YES ☐   **NO** ☐

7) Have you suffered any miscarriage?
YES ☐   **NO** ☐

8) Have you lost any child at birth?
YES ☐   **NO** ☐

9) Is there anything you want to tell us that will help in deciding what faith clinic you need to attend.? (Write on a separate sheet of paper if necessary.)
YES ☐   **NO** ☐

Mail to:
Veronica Anusionwu, The Lords Word On Healing Ministries PO BOX 24604, London E2 9XA

HE LORD'S WORD ON HEALING MINISTRIES

Covenant Partners Form

Dear, partner,

God has called me to bring the Healing Gospel of Jesus to the world. To accomplish this vision I am going to need Faith Covenant Partners. I have prayed that the Lord will send me faithful men and women who will stand with me both financially and spiritually to fulfil this vision. If God is laying it on your heart to partnership with me please respond now.

As a covenant partner I and my prayer team will pray for you every day, will stand with you in faith whenever you need us.

In return I will expect you to sow seed monthly into this ministry or as the spirit of God leads you. Pray for me and my staff as the Spirit of God leads you.

When you sow into the work of God the Bible promises you these benefits: **Protection** (Mal:3 10-11) . **Favour** (Luke 6:38). **Fianacial prosperity** (Deut :8 18).

Please complete this response form and return it to me today.
If you have a prayer request please send it on a seperate sheet of paper.

Name: _____

Address: _____

_____

_____

Mail to:
Veronica Anusionwu: The Lords Word On Healing Ministries PO BOX 24604, London E2 9XA